P9-DHM-819

GET READY TO ENERGIZE YOUR LIFE . . .
. . . . STARTING NOW!

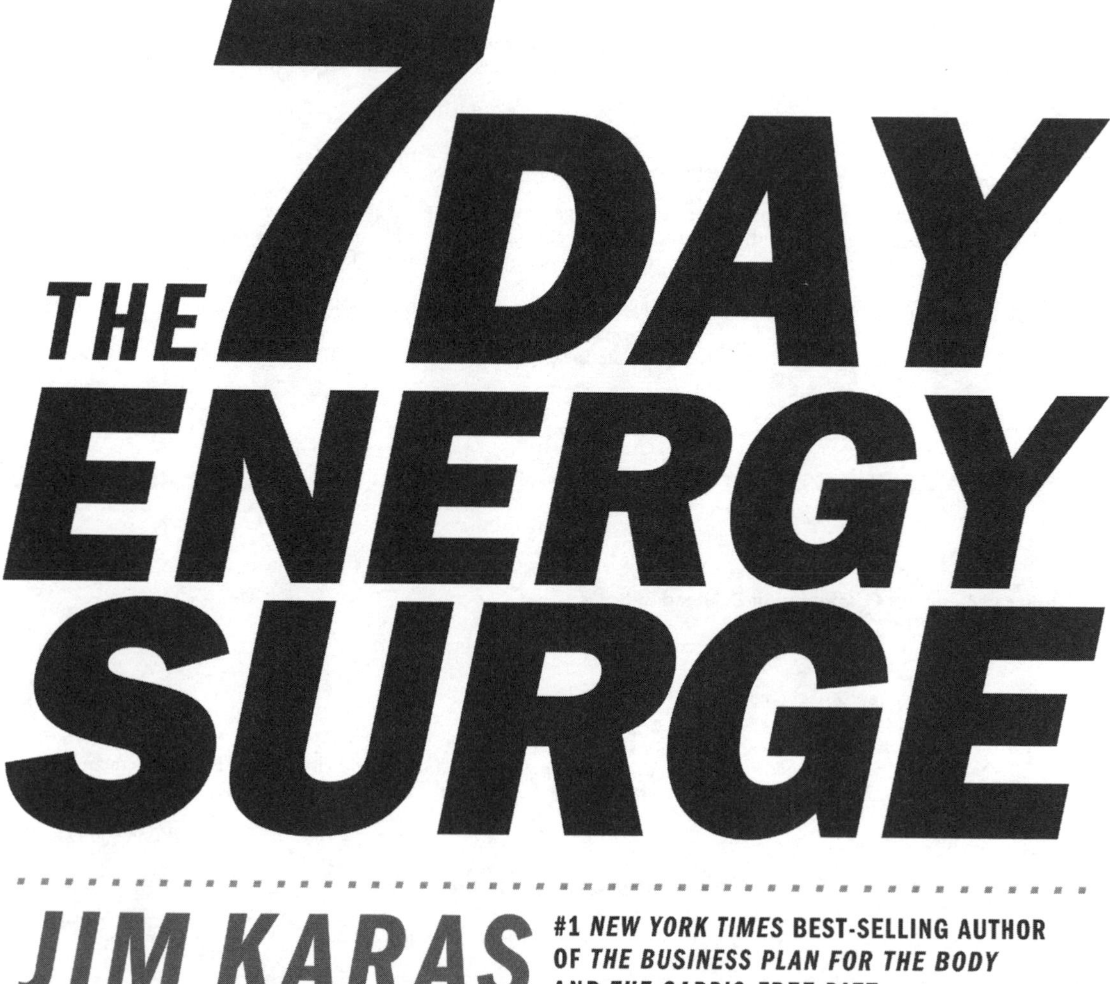

THE 7 DAY ENERGY SURGE

JIM KARAS

#1 *NEW YORK TIMES* BEST-SELLING AUTHOR OF *THE BUSINESS PLAN FOR THE BODY* AND *THE CARDIO-FREE DIET*

WITH CYNTHIA COSTAS COHEN, MFT

Rodale books may be purchased for business or promotional use or for special sales.
For information, please write to:
Special Markets Department, Rodale Inc., 733 Third Avenue, New York, NY 10017

Printed in the United States of America
Rodale Inc. makes every effort to use acid-free ♾, recycled paper ♲.

Photographs by Beth Bischoff

Library of Congress Cataloging-in-Publication Data

Karas, Jim.
The 7-day energy surge / by Jim Karas ; with Cynthia Costas Cohen.
p. cm.
Includes bibliographical references and index.
ISBN-13 978-1-60529-880-1 hardcover
ISBN-10 1-60529-880-8 hardcover
1. Weight training–Therapeutic use. 2. Yoga–Therapeutic use. 3. Physical fitness. 4. Energy medicine. 5. Detoxification (Health) I. Cohen, Cynthia Costas. II. Title. III. Title: Seven-day energy surge.
RM725.K37 2009
613.7'13–dc22 2009003549

Distributed to the trade by Macmillan

2 4 6 8 10 9 7 5 3 1 hardcover

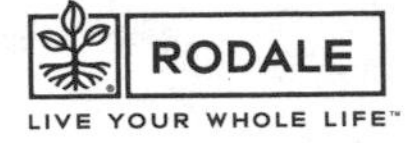

We inspire and enable people to improve their lives and the world around them

For more of our products visit **rodalestore.com** or call 800-848-4735

To Olivia and Evan

ACKNOWLEDGMENTS

First I would like to thank my team in Chicago and New York. When I started as a personal trainer on my own back in 1987, I never envisioned building a firm like ours. Now, 22 years later, I am so very proud of my team of trainers, and want to give a special shout-out to Phil Chung, who leads them with patience, honesty, and trust and is truly an exceptional human being; there is no one to whom I would trust my company more freely or with more confidence.

Then I would like to thank my kids. Olivia, I've said this before, but life has never been the same since the day you popped out . . . and turned . . . and looked right at me. You will always be my baby girl and I love your drive, even at this early age, to be a good friend, a loving sister (well, some of the time) and an amazing, focused athlete. Don't ever lose that and always know that Daddy loves you.

Evan, my creative little man, you must always remember that in your big head, you have an even bigger brain and in your body, you have an incredible warm, loving heart. You are such a gifted artist and I may have to use some of the proceeds of this book to soon rent a warehouse for your original work. Keep laughing, keep loving, and always be true to who you are meant to be.

Finally, to my collaborator, Cynthia, who brought tremendous knowledge, research, experience, and humor, not to mention the endnotes (they almost put me in an institution) to this book. And to her husband, the brilliant writer, director, and producer Larry Cohen, who allowed me to camp out in his home and sequester all of her time and *energy*. Cynthia, you are the sister I never had but always wished for. I don't know what my life would be like without you, but I do know that if I were not in yours, your weight would be up a solid 30 pounds!

CONTENTS

PART I: THE 10 COMPONENTS OF ENERGY

PART II: THE 7-DAY ENERGY SURGE PLAN

INTRODUCTION

WHAT IS ENERGY?

Energy—the capacity of a physical system to do work

Did you know that—

How much you weigh

What you eat and drink

Whether or not you exercise

How well you breathe

The quality and quantity of your sleep

The types of thoughts you entertain

How you deal with stress

The music you listen to

And whether you have had sex recently

—all affect your energy today?

Does this sound familiar? You start your day in a groggy haze as you slap the snooze button three or four times. Then, just getting out of bed (a painful thought) and ready for the day is exhausting. By the time it's 10:00–a.m.–you are dying to take your *first* nap. You practically fall asleep at the wheel, experience brain fog most of the day, and find yourself dozing off during meetings or at your kid's soccer practice.

Then, to make matters worse, you eat the wrong foods at the wrong time (donut anyone?), don't even consider exercise (sorry, yawning doesn't count), never drink a sip of water (unless you have a headache and pop a pill), get on the caffeine *and* sugar highway (I'll take a Coke, a latte, *and* a Red Bull), barely breathe, berate yourself (and possibly your mate) for the past (oh, if you only knew!), live in constant fear of a dreaded future (I'm doomed), and then wonder, "What's wrong with me? I feel horrible and wiped out all the time."

Or you may feel like you have a lot of energy when you're at work and responding to rapid-fire requests from your manager, constant complaints from your customers, and other daily crises, but then you can barely summon the energy to pet the dog or say hello to your kids when you get home. All you can think of is shoveling some food into your mouth and getting to bed, but then once you do, your mind is racing with thoughts of all the things you didn't get done today and won't get a chance to do tomorrow.

You feel that way as a result of BAD habits that annihilate the *capacity of your physical system to do work*—also known as your ENERGY. You know instinctively that these habits are harmful, but hey, at this point, it's routine.

Over the next seven days, I am going to give you a very detailed plan to get you out of your current, downward energy death spiral and into a new, upward-surging "life spiral." It's never too late. If you follow these simple steps, you will instantly be on the path to lasting energy even beyond your wildest dreams—with no corresponding crash (hint—go drink a big glass of cold, sparkling water, then come back and keep reading). Sound too good to be true? I tested this program with real clients with real, busy lives, all of whom felt that the program helped them eat healthier, exercise more, sleep better, and have more energy when they needed it. You'll hear from them directly throughout the book, giving tips on how you can make the 7-Day Energy Surge work for *you*.

You may be wondering, what makes me an *energy expert*? Well, for the past 23 years, I have been called a lot of things (many I can't mention here), such as personal fitness trainer, weight loss expert, food police, life coach, and "The Commander," but none of them felt quite right (well, "The Commander" came close).

I started my career in the weight loss and fitness business back in 1986. Prior to that, I was working as a private portfolio manager, because I had graduated from the Wharton School of Business with a BS in economics. Every Saturday, I used to take a high-impact aerobics class to try to knock off some weight (FYI—it didn't work). And yes, I was a chubber until I learned the smart way to lose the pounds for good (to be shared later).

One Saturday morning, the teacher no-showed for the 8:00 a.m. class, leaving about 100 of us "calorically challenged" members standing around. At 8:15, I surprised myself by blurting out, "Look, if someone can find the music tape, I'll teach," because I had memorized the routine (just so we are clear, you should *never* perform a memorized exercise routine!).

After the 8:00 class, the teacher again no-showed for the 9:00, so I taught that one as well. Afterward, the manager of the club waved me over and said, "Want a job?"

In my best Whartonian manner, I asked, "I don't know. What's your best offer?"

"You get a free membership and $4 an hour," he replied.

I said, "Sold!"

From there, I quickly moved to a swankier, downtown club (for $18 an hour, and that's a 450 percent increase in pay in a VERY short period of time–see, I did use my economics degree) and was approached by my first client, Janet, who asked me to be her personal fitness trainer and offered me $30 an hour. Once again, my reply was, "Sold!"

When I taught a big class, even if I was stressed, rushed, and tired, the moment I put on the music and was feeding on the group energy, I was pumped and ready to go. But when I used to show up to train people one-on-one, I was the sole energy source and it was exhausting.

I quickly realized that I had to crank up my energy. Starting at 4:30 a.m. and training eight to 10 clients a day, seven days a week, in their homes, offices, or private exercise facilities was daunting. It hit me over the head that I had better get a lot of sleep, and often that meant a combination of sleep at night and naps (yes, they were plural at times) to stay at optimal energy output. Ditto with my food and drink, so I planned and packed what I would bring with me.

Breathing was a HUGE part of how I felt, and I would sometimes stand in front of a client's door and just breathe for a minute or two, which also helped clear my mind so that I would give this client my undivided attention. The music I played in my car, on my Walkman (yes, I'm that old), and sometimes in the client's home helped pump me up *and* minimize stress, which was high, given many of my high-profile, demanding clients.

So here I was "on the job," having to learn the balancing act between energy input and energy output. In the meantime, of course, life continued to throw me energy challenges. Twelve years ago, I became a father–trust me, having a baby in the house is a MAJOR factor affecting your energy–and I quickly had to learn how to manage increased demands on my time and energy. Eight years ago, I opened my second personal-fitness training firm in New York, in addition to one in Chicago, and embarked upon a worldwide speaking career that split my energy among more cities than I can count. Then 3 years ago, I got divorced and became "Mr. Mom" more than 50 percent of the time. Talk about another MAJOR demand on my energy that required me to "tweak" my plan once again.

I'm not here to say that these changes were easy, but now I'm a happier, more productive employer, friend, father, and human being. My life is in better balance, and because of that my energy is soaring; it's pouring out of me like never before, and it's truly one of the most intoxicating, natural experiences I've ever had.

In addition to constantly manipulating my own energy equation, I've frequently heard clients tell me that, sure, they liked the way they looked (which generally was terrific), but what really sold them on my plan was the noticeable cascade of energy. Diane Sawyer was one of my first clients to make this connection, which occurred while she was getting up at insane hours to host *Good Morning America*.

I also found that many people had soured on weight loss and fitness programs because they had tried to tackle these issues in the past without much success. I use the term *the buy-in* to determine what will get a potential client to ultimately make the decision to work with one of my team. The more I emphasized "energy" as "the buy-in," the more clients became animated and excited about getting on the plan. That response is what led me to push energy more and more as the ultimate goal and let improved health, weight loss, reduced stress, more effective sleep, etc., follow. That's how the idea for this book was born.

While conceptualizing, researching, and writing this book, I had countless conversations with my very best friend, Cynthia Costas Cohen. Cynthia is a licensed marriage and family therapist (MFT) in addition to being certified by the American Society of Clinical Hypnosis. She has a prominent clientele in Beverly Hills, which includes major celebrities, and it pisses me off that she won't share a single name. In addition, she spends much of her time doing pro bono work for the far less fortunate at a community clinic.

Cynthia directed me to a tremendous body of research, shared her own personal experiences, and taught me techniques that she has successfully used with her patients to enhance energy and well-being. I realized that I needed her collaboration with this endeavor, and her contribution is amazing and critical to a successful surge. Stay tuned, as you will hear directly from Cynthia in certain chapters in a shaded box.

As you go through this 7-day program, you will achieve realistic changes and goals, and each accomplishment will translate into more and more healthy, positive energy. I want you to remember this saying throughout the book:

Accomplishment Creates Energy

You know how great it feels to accomplish something good–giving a terrific presentation, planning a special dinner, or making a commitment to exercise and actually following through with it. I remember the first time I added more memory to my computer. Wow, everything ran faster and more efficiently and I accomplished so much more when I booted up. Now think of your mind and body working faster and more efficiently as you build energy momentum. Once again, energy is truly an exquisite, intoxicating, natural drug, and *you* control it.

Get ready for the 7-Day Energy Surge. It starts now. In no time, you will possess a huge bank of enriching energy. Oh, and this program will also help you lose weight, look great, flatten your abs, lift your butt, breathe efficiently, stall the aging process, have great sex, achieve peace of mind, and feel better than you ever have before.

Hope you don't mind!

HOW TO USE THIS BOOK

THE BALANCE OF ENERGY EQUATION

Let me introduce you to the Balance of Energy Equation:

Body Weight +/–

Calories In (Food *and* Liquids) +/–

Calories Out (Activity, Exercise, *and* Metabolism) +/–

Breathing +/–

Sleep +/–

Mind-set +/–

Stress +/–

Music +/–

Sex =

Energy

Successfully manipulating this equation is the key to optimal energy.

Notice that it's one equation and all the variables work together. When most people think about cultivating energy, they may *just* work on eating, *just* start to exercise, *just* improve sleep habits, or *just* try to reduce stress. Sure, doing *something* is better than nothing, but the key is to simultaneously chip away at all the elements that affect energy.

I bet the majority of you are doing a lot of smart things to enhance your energy, and then doing one or two things that are not so smart (the classic trifecta is sleep deprivation, dehydration, and raging stress), and that negates any positive energy initiatives. Do not let that happen.

Are all the variables equally important? I have to say yes. The key to this energy surge is balance. Think about building a house of cards. Does each and every card have to be in the right place to support the entire structure? Yes. Are they equally important? Yes. What happens when just one card gets out of balance? Generally, the structure collapses.

Now take the 7-Day Energy Surge Quiz to determine your overall energy level and the components you need to focus on most.

7-Day Energy Surge Quiz

1. I wake up every morning feeling:

1—awful

2—that I need another hour of sleep, at least

3—pretty much the same, not rested but not wiped out

4—ready to start the day with a cup of coffee

5—energized

2. My body weight is:

1—terrible, because I have gained a lot of weight and have kept it on

2—pretty bad, because I struggle and can't stop losing and gaining the same weight

3—what it has been for a long time, higher than I want but not horrible

4—I recently started a weight loss plan and have taken off ______ pounds

5—pretty close to my ideal weight

3. My eating habits are:

1—terrible, because I just can't stop overeating all the time

2—good during the day but not so good on the evenings and weekends

3—about the same as they have been for a long time, up and down—I just can't get in a healthy and consistent routine for more than a day or two

4—better than they have been in a long time, because I am making more careful choices and have eliminated a lot of the junk

5—I'm making very good choices and can feel the difference in my weight and my energy levels

4. My drinking habits are:

1—terrible, because I am not drinking water and drink too much coffee, juice, soda, sports drinks, and alcohol

2—not so, so bad, but I don't drink more than two glasses of water and am still at about five+ cups of coffee a day

3—somewhat routine, because I do fill my 32-ounce water bottle once a day (and finish it) and have cut back on drinking wine, with the exception of the weekends

4—much better, because I limit myself to two cups of coffee a day, more tea, less alcohol, and at least 50 ounces of water a day

5—really good, because I only have one cup of coffee first thing in the morning, and drink more tea and at least 75 to 80 ounces of water a day. I've also cut my alcohol down to four total glasses of wine a week.

5. My exercise habits are:

1—terrible, because I haven't exercised consistently in years

2—I try to walk most places, but don't usually do it except on the weekends

3—I walk to and from my bus stop/train station/office from my garage every day and do a workout in my home or gym about once a week

4—I get in two 45-minute workouts a week and meet a friend to walk for an hour every Saturday

5—I consistently get in three or four 30-minute workouts a week and do a combination of strength training and aerobics

6. My breathing habits are:

1—I'm barely breathing, because my chest and diaphragm hardly move and I never think about it

2 –I breathe shallowly but every now and then I sigh or yawn

3—my chest and shoulders slightly go up with each breath and every now and then I try to take a few deeper breaths

4—with each breath, my chest expands and occasionally my belly fills—every hour or so I check in with my breath

5—with each breath, my belly fills up with air and flows into my lungs and I am mindful and present

7. My sleeping habits are:

1—terrible, because I only sleep 4 or 5 hours a night and get up and go to bed at all different times

2—pretty bad, because I only sleep 5 or 6 hours a night and frequently awaken in the middle of the night

3—okay, because I sleep between 6 and 7 hours a night, but I almost always wish I had another hour in the morning to sleep and have to use an alarm clock and hit the snooze button repeatedly. I also frequently try to catch up on sleep on the weekend.

4—better, because I sleep between 7 and 8 hours five nights a week and around 6 or 7 the other two—I only have to use an alarm about 50 percent of the time

5—great, because I sleep between 7 and 8 hours every night, always go to bed and get up within the same 30-minute time period, and rarely if ever have to use an alarm

8. My overall mind-set is:

1—negative, because I dwell far too much on the past

2—generally down, but I do try to minimize past failures

3—okay; I have good and bad days, and they balance out in the long run

4—upbeat, because I can usually talk myself out of a death spiral and try to live and look at the glass as half full rather than half empty

5—very up and people comment that my positive attitude makes me fun to be around

9. My stress levels are:

1—out of control, because I live in a state of overwhelming stress

2—pretty high during the week but somewhat better on the weekends

3—up and down, depending on the day and the situation

4—generally good, with an occasional dip due to family, work, relationship, kids, or illness, either my own or affecting someone I care a great deal about

5—under complete control, because I know the warning signs when I am getting overly stressed out and have the coping skills to alleviate it

10. I listen to music:

1—almost never

2—sometimes when I am in my car

3—on the weekends when I am working around the house and remember to put something on

4—most nights when I get home from work/my day with the kids and need to relax

5—all the time, in the morning, when I work out, at my office or computer, and at night, when it's time to wind down

11. I have sex with a partner:

1—almost never

2—maybe once every other month

3—maybe once a month

4—once a week

5—more than once a week

12. I have sex, um, with myself:

1—almost never

2—once every 2 weeks

3—once every week

4—two or three times a week

5—more than four times a week (go for it!)

Now, tally up your score, which will place you in one of the following three categories:

- Low Energy = 0 to 20
- Moderate Energy = 21 to 39
- High Energy = 40 to 60

Key:

- If you fall into the Low Energy category, then you clearly have a lot of work to do. Don't let that discourage you, and be happy that you have the book in your hands and are ready to accept the challenge. Plus, let's face it, your score can only go up if you follow the guidelines set forth, so go for it.
- If you fall into the Moderate Energy category, then you are already on the road to the surge. You probably have been consciously making smarter energy choices, but now you need the structure of this book to make those choices more effective.
- If you are in the High Energy category, you are doing really, really well and will only require micro adjustments. It's time for fine-tuning and thinking about the difference between a good presentation and a great one. That's your mission.

Note: You will be asked to take this quiz again at the end of the 7-Day Energy Surge, so please keep a record of your starting score. If you follow the plan wholeheartedly, I promise you will see an improvement in your scores! All of our testers improved their energy scores by an average of 8 points; one woman experienced a jump of 11.

You may notice that your scores are lopsided, with a lot of 4s and 5s, but some 1s and 2s that knocked your total energy score down. Pay special attention to the components that correspond to the low scores. Although I want you to read the book in order, I urge you to reread those sections that correspond to the components that require the most attention and perform each of the exercises outlined.

And please don't skip sections! Even if you scored 5s in a few areas and feel as if you've mastered those variables, you can always fine-tune how you deal with them, or learn something you can share with others–and helping others percolates *your* energy. So, even though I know you're anxious to dive right in, I urge you to read the whole book first, in order, from cover to cover, to see how certain themes prevail throughout the book and how all the components work together. I promise that it will be a quick read and worth your time! I conceptualized the book so that you first deal with your body, then your mind, and then add music and a satisfying sex life.

Note: You might have a high overall energy score, but frequently feel burned out or drained by the end of a long day. If that's the case, this plan can help you, too! The

7-Day Energy Surge doesn't just rev up your energy; it also keeps you on an even keel so that you don't crash.

Although all of the components affect each other, you will notice that the first three variables of the equation–Body Weight, Calories In, and Calories Out–work especially closely together. If, like the majority of Americans, you've ever been on a diet, you'll know that genetics and biology play a role in your weight and your metabolism. But that doesn't mean you should despair of reaching your ideal body weight! There are a lot of things you can control to affect each of these three variables, and in my plan I'll concentrate on those components–namely, what you eat and drink and how you exercise.

In the next 10 chapters, "baby steps" will be presented to fine-tune your personal balance of energy equation. Although it's unrealistic to think that you will be able to reach your ideal body weight, change all your bad habits, and magically have the life of your dreams in 7 days, research points to the fact that small changes lead to big changes over the long run. Take, for example, Component 10, Sex to *Big* Surge. Can you totally change your sex life in 7 days? Probably not, but can you make wise changes that lead you in the right direction? Absolutely, if you spend a little time and thought on your "sexual energy." It's very much akin to compounding interest; a little bit here and a little bit there equals huge investment (energy) gains.

One final note: This plan starts on a Monday. I have found for most people (myself included) that Monday represents a fresh start and a clean slate. It also gives you the weekend to shop, plan, prepare, and schedule for this 7-day program. Plus, I know from talking to thousands of people that the weekend is the hardest time to stay on *any* plan. By building a solid foundation of energy *momentum* during the week, you will be infinitely better prepared for the challenges of the weekend. Think of Monday as D-Day, or should I say, Energy-Day.

But if you happen to have picked up this book midweek, that doesn't mean you can't get started right away. There are a few things you can do right now to prepare for your energy surge:

1. Take a few deep breaths.

2. Drink a glass of cold water.

What You'll Need for the 7-Day Energy Surge

- SPRI StrengthCord braided tubing with door attachment
- scale
- mattress less than 10 years old that supports your back
- pillows less than 1 year old that support your neck
- sheets that are soft, cool, and comfortable
- earplugs
- sleep mask
- snore strips (if your mate snores)
- dim night-light
- pet bed (if you own a pet)
- harmonica or other wind instrument
- stereo, iPod, or other music player

3. Remind yourself of a success you've accomplished in the past.

4. Start a food diary, recording what you eat and when, and how you feel before and after your meal.

5. Collect the equipment you'll need for the 7-Day Energy Surge (see box above). You'll also find more information about the equipment you'll need in the preparation chapter starting on page 184.

And finally, of course, begin reading about the 10 components of energy!

PART I

THE 10 COMPONENTS OF ENERGY

COMPONENT 1

BODY WEIGHT TO SURGE

Being a leader in the weight loss industry allows me to say, hands down, that *nothing* depletes your energy more than excess body weight.

Think about a time when you were lighter, by just a few pounds or more, and complete the following sentence on an index card or a small piece of paper:

"When I was lighter . . ."

Here are some of the responses I have heard over the years:

"I woke up with more energy."
"I was proud that I was taking care of myself and respecting my body."
"I saw that look on my partner's face and my spirits soared."
"I had a more positive aura and got hit on more."
"I didn't insist on 'lights off' during sex."

Like a teeter-totter, the moment the weight goes down you will immediately feel your energy bubble up. Each and every pound makes a difference, so don't sit back and say, "I have 50-plus pounds to lose. Ugh, it'll take forever." No, no, no, every pound makes a difference, so consider each one lost a personal victory.

Keep your written responses with you at all times, especially when nearing what I refer to as the "Danger Zone," that is, the weekend. Come on, Friday night is generally the beginning of the weekend eating frenzy (that's why we started this plan on Monday, remember?), but not the weekend of your 7-Day Energy Surge; the support of your written word will help keep you motivated, and you should use it as each subsequent weekend approaches. Ditto for the holidays!

When you are lighter, you will feel proud and confident *and* get more accomplished on a daily basis. Weighing less will almost always translate into improved health. This means fewer aches and pains, fewer sick days, fewer doctor visits, less time waiting in line to fill prescriptions, etc., etc., etc., and more oomph–and energy–for work, family, friends, pets, and fun. Are you getting the point?

Research backs this up. A study reported in the *Journal of Occupational and Environmental Medicine* found that as body mass index (BMI) increased, so did the number of sick days, because being overweight is so clearly the cause of numerous debilitating illnesses, such as diabetes, sleep apnea, and heart disease. By lowering your body weight, you immediately lower the risk of these diseases and increase your energy potential.[1] Plus, losing weight makes you feel sexy. If you think that you have to be in *Vogue* or *Men's Health* shape to have more sex, then read on. Duke University's Martin Binks found that *just* a 10 percent weight loss significantly improved the sex lives of men and women. Sexual satisfaction peaked at 12 percent weight loss; more loss than that was insignificant.[2] With more sex comes more happy endorphin hormones circulating in your system (where do you think the term *afterglow* came from?), which in turn boosts libido, reduces stress, and, let's face it, puts you in a pretty cheery mood. It's a great, positive "life spiral" for igniting energy (much, much more on sex and energy in Component 10).

If you are presently overweight, lowering your body weight is essential to the energy surge and is something you can start on TODAY. Now, of course, your body weight is going to be a function of what you eat and drink, how you exercise, your sleep patterns, your breathing, your stress level, your mind-set, how much you listen to music, and so on, but a few additional tips are helpful:

BUY A SCALE

Now, now, now, don't panic. Just the *thought* of the scale sends most people running, but the scale is actually your friend. Research from both Brown University Medical School and the University of Minnesota conclusively demonstrated that the more often you weigh yourself, the less you weigh.[3, 4] Repeat that with me a moment:

"The more you weigh, the less you'll weigh."

Plus, those who did not get on the scale GAINED weight in both studies.

UNDERSTAND THAT 3,500 CALORIES EQUALS ONE POUND

Simply put, eat 3,500 more calories than your body requires and you will gain a pound. Expend 3,500 more calories through metabolism and activity than you consume and you'll lose a pound. It's all math, and simple math at that.

SET A REALISTIC GOAL

Because you now know that 3,500 calories equal 1 pound, you have to work the numbers. In these first 7 days, I do all the work for you, but if you want to lose 1 pound a week in the future, eat 500 *fewer* calories a day than your body requires. After 7 days, that 500-calorie deficit will equal 1 pound lost (500×7 days $= 3{,}500$). If you want to lose 2 pounds in 1 week, then eat 1,000 fewer calories each day.

To find out how many calories you require to maintain your current weight, fill in the following equation, which will give you the amount of calories you presently require to maintain your weight, without activity:

Women: resting metabolic rate = 655 + (4.35 × weight in pounds) + (4.7 × height in inches) – (4.7 × age in years)

Men: resting metabolic rate = 66 + (6.23 × weight in pounds) + (12.7 × height in inches) – (6.8 × age in years)

Take that number and multiply it by one of the following numbers:

Activity Factor	Category	Definition
1.2	Sedentary	Little or no exercise and desk job
1.375	Lightly Active	Light exercise 1 to 3 days a week
1.55	Moderately Active	Moderate exercise 3 to 5 days a week
1.725	Very Active	Hard exercise 6 to 7 days a week
1.9	Extremely Active	Hard daily exercise and physical job

From this final number, you determine how many calories you want to subtract. If you don't want to figure out these numbers on your own, then go to www.jimkaras.com and you will find the metabolic rate calculator on the site.

In the beginning phase of this plan, I would say that 3 to 4 pounds a week for women and 4 to 5 for men is realistic because you are releasing body fat *and* bloating water weight while you are cleansing your system. After the "honeymoon" phase (approximately 2 to 3 weeks), women can expect a 1- to 2-pound loss and men a 2- to 3-pound loss per week.

A Word from Our Testers

"I wasn't looking to lose weight, but I am down 4 pounds already. I have never weighed less—even when marathon training!"

—Andrew M., age 41

GET OUT YOUR JEANS

I know, I know, they probably aren't comfy, but they will be soon. You're wearing them on Saturday and Sunday of your designated surge week because, let's face it, jeans don't lie. If they are loose, that means the scale or your inches or both are down. If they feel the same way they did last week, then there's proof that you haven't really been on the plan.

FIND OR BUY THE SMALLEST PLATES AND GLASSES

There is a whole body of knowledge that proves that the smaller the plate, bowl, or glass, the less you will eat or drink. Quick, take a look in your kitchen cabinets and tell me: How big is your everyday china and glassware? Research shows that everything is just getting bigger and bigger, so we keep piling it on to fill the plate. Stop it. Here is a strategy–use salad plates for your main course, eat, then wait 15 minutes and decide whether you want another helping. Odds are, you will opt out, because it takes about 15 to 20 minutes for you to finally feel full.

KEEP A FOOD DIARY

On the Saturday and Sunday before your 7-Day Energy Surge, write down everything you eat *as* you eat it. Don't wait until the end of the day and fake it. I coined the phrase "You Bite It, You Write It" in *O, The Oprah Magazine*; keeping a food diary, even for just these 2 days, is an invaluable tool for losing weight and bumping up your energy, because it serves two specific purposes:

1. You see every bite in writing. People always look me straight in the eye and say, "I'm not overeating," only to discover a few days later, when faced with the actual numbers, that they are taking undisclosed and undeserved liberties in a big way.

2. It helps you self-monitor. For example, while walking down the aisle of Whole Foods (referred to as "Whole Paycheck" in my office–but their stuff *is* great), it's a virtual

minefield of free samples every 3 feet–tidbits of cheese, seaweed candy, turkey tofu, etc. Approaching each station, you might be asking yourself, "Do I, don't I, do I, don't I . . . ?" ideally followed by, "Oh forget it. I'm really not that hungry and I don't want to have to write it down." Mindless, excessive eating significantly depletes energy because all of your body's resources go into digesting the additional food.

The National Weight Control Registry agrees with my advice. This group represents individuals who successfully kept 30 pounds off for at least a year, and the vast majority of them diligently kept a food diary.[5]

GET RID OF WEIGHT LOSS GIMMICKS THAT DIDN'T WORK

Purge yourself of all the misinformation you have ever read, heard, or believed with regard to weight loss. If any of it really worked, you wouldn't be reading this chapter. Throw out all your old weight loss gizmos, books, ThighMaster (which injured some people), Jane Fonda's videotapes, and anything lying around the house that hasn't worked and only adds clutter and confusion to your ultimate goal. Clutter and confusion is energy leeching–big time! If you don't believe me, tell me how you feel every time you open that closet filled with sh&^%$#t.

GO PUBLIC

In my first book, the #1 *New York Times* bestseller, *The Business Plan for the Body*, I used the analogy of a business plan and applied it to weight loss. One of the most popular chapters was called "Go Public." In it, I advised readers to tell everyone, and I mean everyone, that they were going to successfully lose weight and feel great; I beg you to do the same. If you don't embrace that public declaration, then you must be considering failing privately.

GET A WEIGHT LOSS BUDDY

I want you to invite someone to exercise with you on Saturday or Sunday, because the weekend is easier to schedule. Researchers at the University of Pittsburgh School of Medicine found that after 10 months, 66 percent of those with a bud kept their weight off, versus 24 percent who went at it alone.[6] That's a HUGE difference, so take a moment and decide who would be your ideal, supportive partner. Make the call, book it, and do it!

Your buddy may or may not be on this same plan with you, but it should be someone you would enjoy working out or spending time with. Consider acquiring two sets of the SPRI exercise tubing and door attachments that you will be using in the exercise plan outlined in Component 4 so that you can exercise side-by-side.

SCHEDULE A COMPREHENSIVE PHYSICAL IF YOU HAVEN'T HAD ONE IN THE PAST YEAR

You are about to embark on a program to optimize energy, and you therefore need as much data as possible. I also want you to get clearance to exercise if you have had past medical issues.

At the very least, you need to get the following tests:

- Cholesterol
- Blood pressure
- Fasting blood sugar
- Bone density, especially for postmenopausal women
- Thyroid panel blood test
- Vitamin D level (*Note:* According to Michael F. Holick, PhD, MD, one-half of all Americans are chronically deprived of vitamin D.)[7]

Your physician should determine what else is relevant, and please, make it a point to discuss every medication and supplement that you are on. Many people don't realize that some of their medications and supplements, or even certain foods, counteract the benefits of some medications, and there are also many prescriptions that cause weight gain. These "weight positive" medications include those for high blood pressure, diabetes, heart conditions, inflammation, and depression, to name a few.

Two-thirds of the American population is overweight or obese. Therefore, the majority of you will be working on this body weight issue. Many of the sections in this book, such as what to eat and drink, and how to exercise and sleep, deal directly or indirectly with body weight, but be sure to follow the specific directions outlined in this section. Trust me, excess body weight is a true energy *extinguisher* and is something that you can begin to change immediately.

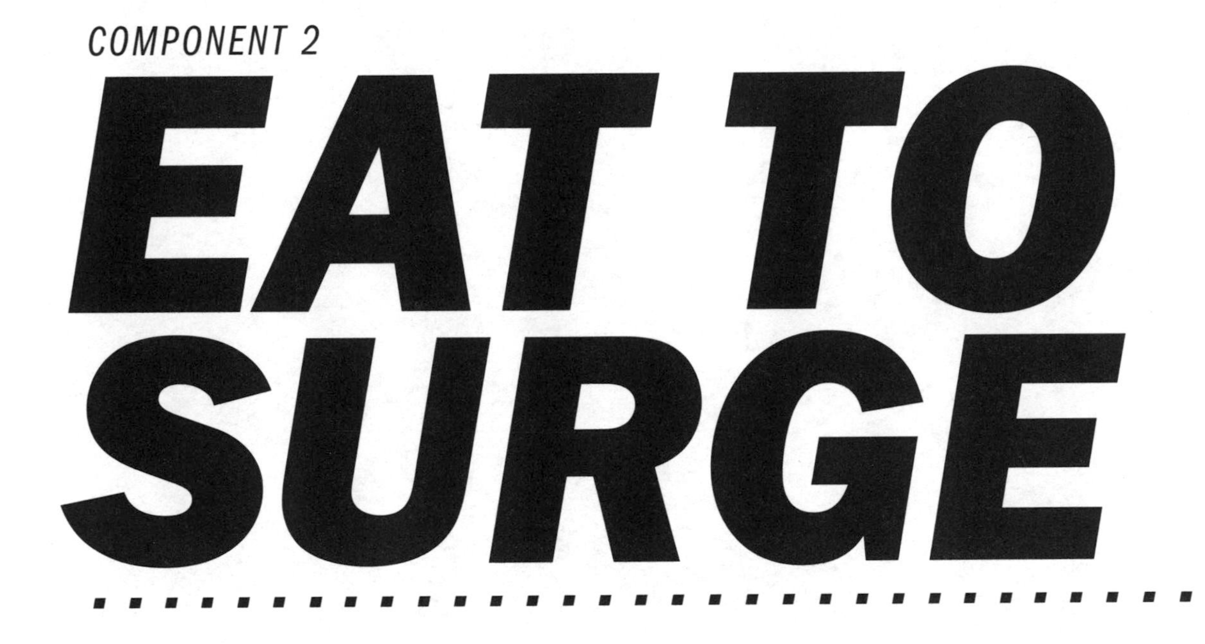
COMPONENT 2
EAT TO
SURGE

In this chapter, we are going to look at your "Calories In" and concentrate specifically on food, because I will cover liquids in the next chapter.

In the next three components, I will follow a template that categorizes behaviors or foods and drinks according to how much of them you want to allow. Your 7-Day Energy Surge plan will automatically regulate these actions and foods, but keep these guidelines in mind past these 7 days and watch your energy soar.

Behaviors You Should Perform More Of

- ☐ Count calories
- ☐ Add a little bit of protein to every meal
- ☐ Eat lots of fruits and vegetables
- ☐ Consume whole wheat or whole grain carbohydrates
- ☐ Eat before and after each workout
- ☐ Follow a 1,200-calorie eating plan
- ☐ Always have balsamic vinegar or fresh lemon or lime nearby
- ☐ Prepare good-smelling foods

Foods You Should Consume Sparingly

- ☐ Olive oil
- ☐ Salad dressing
- ☐ Avocado
- ☐ Legumes

Behaviors You Should Avoid

- ☐ Skipping breakfast
- ☐ Waiting too long between meals or snacks
- ☐ Driving on the "Sugar Highway"
- ☐ Consuming too many calories
- ☐ Overeating on the weekends
- ☐ Eating Caesar salad
- ☐ Saddling up to fast food

BEHAVIORS YOU SHOULD PERFORM MORE OF

COUNT CALORIES

Okay, we won't call it counting calories; we'll call it improving your "caloric awareness." Caloric awareness is the only way to successfully lose weight AND stay on a plan that makes sense for the long run. For your 7-Day Energy Surge, I do all the counting, portion control, and work for you, so don't panic. It's after that 7-day period that you have to do more of the work to reverse the overeating trend and lose weight. If it's easier, you may continue to eat the 7-day plan indefinitely.

To truly understand and estimate the calories of what you are putting into your mouth, you need to read labels. Two essential lines are:

- Calories per serving
- Servings per container

Favorite story–an overweight and out-of-shape CEO in Chicago worked with my team of trainers and he and I would also periodically meet to review his diet. One day, he listed "ice cream" at the end of his food diary and wrote down "150 calories"–a true red flag.

"What did you eat?" I asked.

"Ice cream," he replied.

Again I asked, "What did you eat?"

"Ice cream," he replied louder.

Exasperated, I finally shouted, "Did you eat the whole container?"

"Of course I did!"

That, for the record, is 150 calories times 4, because there are four servings per container for a grand total of 600 calories of ice cream.

Keep in mind, a single, one-half cup serving of most popular ice cream brands would fill half a baseball, NOT a softball–NOT a football. That's not a whole lotta food; that's not a whole lotta fun. Some "designer" ice creams are close to 350 calories per serving, which translates into 1,400 calories for the whole container. Ouch!

Read your labels!

ADD A LITTLE BIT OF PROTEIN TO EVERY MEAL

Protein is the most difficult food for your body to digest and will therefore enable you to stay full longer. Common sources of protein include:

- Animal protein, such as beef, chicken, turkey, and fish. Ideally, I want you to choose the leanest animal protein, such as boneless, skinless chicken or turkey. Red meat is fine in a portion-controlled manner, and filet is one of your best choices. Fish is generally great (I love salmon), but do be careful with certain types, such as tuna, which may be high in mercury. Also, canned tuna is high in sodium, so I suggest that you place it in a strainer and run cold water over it to eliminate some of it. And don't even think about eating the skin on the chicken or turkey, because the skin is like candle wax in your bloodstream and is loaded with fat, cholesterol, calories, and toxins.
- Legumes, such as any kind of beans (chickpeas, black beans, kidney beans, edamame, and soybeans), peas, lentils, and nuts. Although they are a great source of protein, they are being placed in the "Consume Sparingly" category because they can quickly add up in calories.
- Dairy, such as yogurt, cottage cheese, and certain cheeses that possess less fat. Low-fat dairy is also a terrific source of calcium, which is critical to bone health as both women and men age. I generally don't recommend fat-free products, because they don't keep you satisfied as long. But dairy is an exception. Because the "real" thing is very high in calories and cholesterol, please keep to the 1 and 2 percent varieties.

Protein is made up of amino acids. Think of protein as a pearl necklace and the individual pearls as amino acids. When you ingest protein, the stomach breaks the necklace apart and puts it back together for use in the human body. This act of breaking it apart and putting it back together takes a long time in the stomach, which is why you stay full longer.

Note: Further research also proves that the more protein you consume, the more lean muscle tissue you *preserve* on a restricted calorie diet. A University of Illinois study found that eating high-quality protein helped overweight women maintain muscle mass and reduce body fat during weight loss.[3]

Low-Fat Dairy and Weight Loss

There is research that claims that calcium-rich dairy accelerates weight loss. The findings were first uncovered by Dr. Michael Zemel from the University of Tennessee while examining how calcium-rich dairy reduced blood pressure. Not only did the participants lower their pressure, but they also each lost approximately 11 pounds while the control group, eating the same amount of calories, didn't.

Zemel then conducted a 24-week clinical trial of approximately 30 overweight adults and placed them all on a low-calorie diet and divided them into three groups:

1. Those who only consumed a 400- to 500-mg calcium supplement
2. Those who only consumed an 800 mg supplement
3. Those who consumed 1,200 to 1,300 mg of calcium from low-fat dairy products

After the 24 weeks, the results showed that, as a percentage of body weight:

1. The low-calcium-supplement group lost 6.4 percent, with 20 percent in the abdominal region, a problematic area, because it is so close to your heart that it increases your risk of many diseases.
2. The high-calcium-supplement group lost 7.7 percent.
3. The low-fat dairy consumers lost 10.9 percent, with 66 percent in the abdominal region.[1]

Now, it is important to let you know that Zemel's research was funded by the dairy industry and the makers of Yoplait yogurt, General Mills.

Since then, Harvard School of Public Health analyzed the data from about 20,000 men over a 12-year period and found no correlation between dairy intake and additional weight loss. In another study conducted by Jean Harvey-Berino, chairman of the department of nutrition and food sciences at the University of Vermont, overweight people did not show accelerated weight loss when consuming more dairy.[2]

Although the research is mixed, in my personal experience, I've found that clients who do consume low-fat dairy products often do manage their weight more effectively. I love the taste and find it very satisfying, so I do consume a lot of low-fat dairy products and encourage my staff, readers, viewers, and listeners to do the same.

EAT LOTS OF FRUITS AND VEGETABLES

Fruits and vegetables are essential for optimal energy, reduced body weight, and improved health. They provide many, many other beneficial compounds for the body, in addition to also being a great source of water (more on that in the next component). I fully believe that 50 percent of your daily calories should come from fruits and vegetables. One of the simplest strategies is to include fruit in your breakfast and snacks and make one meal a day a big salad with about 6 ounces of lean protein and very low-calorie dressing. It's easy, it's tasty, and after eating a simple salad, your energy will soar.

I am also a HUGE fan of eating apples before meals or as snacks because:

- They are available year-round.
- They are generally inexpensive (though the organic ones do get a little pricey at times. According to Shopper's Guide to Pesticides in Produce, apples are number two, after peaches, as the most toxic food, so be sure to thoroughly wash the conventionally grown ones).[4]
- They crunch. I have always found that crunchy food is more satisfying.
- They travel easily in your purse, briefcase, glove compartment, or suitcase AND they have been proven to help you eat less.

A study from Penn State found that eating an apple 15 minutes before an all-you-can-eat pasta meal led the participants to consume 15 percent fewer calories.[5] This goes along with another body of research that claims that people eating apples within a 24-hour period are 27 percent less likely to develop metabolic syndrome, a physical condition that includes elevated blood sugar, blood pressure, and cholesterol.[6] Finally, Cornell University researchers fed mice a known carcinogen along with apple extracts. They found that extracts correlating to one, three, or six apples a day reduced cancer rates by 17, 39, and 44 percent respectively; tumors were cut by up to 61 percent.[7]

I urge you to have apples everywhere, on your kitchen counter, desk, conference room table, picnic table, anywhere that you can plainly see them, because we eat with our eyes. The more you see the apples, the more likely you will actually eat one.

And for the record, eat all varieties of apples, because each type possesses potent vitamins that reduce body weight, enhance immunity, slow the aging process, and increase ENERGY!

CONSUME WHOLE WHEAT OR WHOLE GRAIN CARBOHYDRATES

According to the USDA, only 7 percent of Americans get the recommended three servings of whole grains a day.[8] That's shockingly low. In addition, whole wheat and whole grains exit the stomach very *slowly* and gradually release sugar (glucose) into the bloodstream. Therefore, blood sugar levels remain much more constant, which translates into consistent energy. I will go into more detail on this subject later in this section.

Researchers at Penn Sate have shown that consuming more whole grains leads to more abdominal fat loss and a reduction in inflammation linked to that same metabolic syndrome described earlier.

In this study, 50 overweight people were separated into two groups and placed on a calorie-restricted diet–one group consumed only whole grain carbohydrates and the other refined carbohydrates (the white stuff). At the end of the 12-week trial, both groups lost an average of 8 to 11 pounds, but the whole grain group shed more from the abdominal area and experienced a 38 percent decrease in blood levels of C-reactive protein, which is an inflammatory protein linked to an increased risk of diabetes, heart attack, stroke, and high blood pressure. Inflammation is bad, bad, bad for your health and energy. If you can believe it, the C-reactive numbers were similar to people on statins, or cholesterol-lowering drugs, which happen to be the number one most prescribed drug in the United States.[9]

In addition, researchers in the Netherlands found that those eating more whole grains are less likely to be overweight or obese. In fact, they found that with each extra gram of whole grain fiber consumed, the risk of obesity dropped 10 percent for men and 4 percent for women. Those are big numbers PER gram of fiber.[10]

But please, keep the portion of any "wheaty" complex carbs down. Don't eat a 500-calorie, whole wheat bagel and pat yourself on the back for a good choice. Ditto with a

The Connections between Eating, Sleeping, and Sex

Although I will talk all about sleep and sex in Components 6 and 10, scientists at Santa Clara University found that eating better, and specifically reducing blood sugar levels and body weight, resulted in more vivid dreams while sleeping, especially the sexual kind. Upping your consumption of whole grains, fruits, and vegetables may lead to more energizing, exciting deep slumber and possibly some interesting memories when you get up in the morning.[11]

The Power of Fiber

You cannot get enough fiber these days, because it assists you in:

- Staying full
- Lowering cholesterol
- Pushing toxins out of your body
- Reducing inflammation
- Breathing (the latest findings show that 27 grams of fiber a day lead to a larger lung capacity as well as a 15 percent decrease in a chronic lung disease that is very common in our later years).[12] Much more on breathing and energy to come.

I hope it is clear by now that adding more fiber to your diet via fruits, vegetables, legumes, and whole grains results in an energy *explosion*.

huge bowl of whole wheat pasta. You must always be aware of the amount of calories you are consuming. Plus, make sure that the first or second ingredient on the label says "whole wheat" or "whole grain," or it's just brown-colored white stuff.

EAT BEFORE AND AFTER EACH WORKOUT

See, I'm letting you eat, and you probably assumed I would want you to starve. Tricked you! Eating before and after exercise optimizes all the effort you put into each session. You must eat before exercise, because neglecting to do so will lower blood sugar and may lead you to overeat postworkout.

Plus, eating enhances exercise performance. A study from Pennsylvania State University proved that women who had a light meal before their workout were able to go 16 percent longer than those who only had water.[13] A perfect preexercise meal would be a piece of whole wheat toast or fruit, even a small portion of dried fruit, oatmeal (which is ideal), or a bowl of cereal and milk. Now, it's true, if you don't eat before your workout, you may burn more fat, but you may also burn muscle. Not good, so please, eat before you hit the interval strength training.

Note: There has been so much attention given to which fuel source you are using when working out. It does *not* matter whether you are burning fat for fuel, because you must work at a very low intensity for a very long time to accomplish that goal. All that matters is the total amount of calories that you burn during and after the workout, so please, don't worry about which fuel you are using when working out.

Eating postworkout is critical because it provides the building blocks, or amino acids in protein, to optimally begin the muscular repair process (much more on this concept in Component 4). The snacks that I recommend in *The 7-Day Energy Surge* are ideal for this purpose. According to Dr. John Ivy, chairperson of the department of kinesiology and health education at the University of Texas, Austin, by eating the right food immediately (as in no more than 30 minutes after and optimally the moment you finish working out), you will "recover more effectively, work out harder more frequently, increase muscle mass, burn more fat and enhance all the physical adaptations that are happening."[14] I have always noticed that some of the men in the best shape in the locker room are always eating or drinking something the moment they are done. I have been doing that now for a number of years, and I notice a difference in both my results and my energy postworkout.

Research is showing that low-fat milk may be the perfect postexercise drink (more on that in the next chapter), and a British study showed that eating a postworkout snack that is high in protein (as opposed to a sugary drink) burned 21 percent more energy postworkout, because you spend more energy digesting protein than you do carbs.[15]

Another study from Georgia Southern University showed that eating a high-protein, high-fat snack (such as almonds or an egg, which I think are the *perfect* postworkout fuels) increased the afterburn 3½ hours compared to a high-protein, low-fat snack. I will give you a complete description of afterburn in Component 4, Exercise to Surge.[16]

FOLLOW A 1,200-CALORIE EATING PLAN

Part of the reason I am calling this the 7-Day Energy Surge is because I want to drop your calories significantly down to enable you to immediately feel your energy pop. Excessive eating depletes energy, but smart, low-calorie eating increases it. Research shows that 1,200 calories is an acceptable amount that will *not* cause a woman's metabolism to diminish (it's 1,400 for men), so don't be concerned about that happening.[17] In the past, some dieticians and nutritionists were concerned that 1,200 calories may cause a woman's body to go into starvation mode. Similar to when you skip meals, starvation mode causes your metabolism to decline, and that comes as a result of diminished lean muscle tissue. But that has not proved to be true. You also will be performing interval strength training, which will enable you to maintain and increase your calorie-burning lean muscle tissue while on this eating plan. Much more on this in Component 4.

Note: The eating plan you'll find in Part II gives you 1,200 calories a day. Men need to add 200 additional calories a day. This can be accomplished by adding the appropriate portion of the following:

- One serving of fruit, which is 100 calories and defined as one medium-size piece or ½ cup cut up.
- An additional egg–90 calories
- An additional yogurt–generally 100 calories
- 4 additional ounces of grilled chicken–approximately 180 calories
- A few more of the approved ingredients in the 7-Day Eating Surge in a portion-controlled manner

I have purposely balanced the protein, fat, and carbohydrates in this meal plan so that you will not feel hungry. Again, some people in the past have complained of a reduced amount of energy when eating only 1,200 calories, but that had more to do with *what* they were eating than with how many calories they were eating. Clearly, three 400-calorie white bagels a day will *not* lead to a flurry of energy.

After your 7-day plan, if you determine that it is the ideal strategy to continue your surge, you may continue to consume only 1,200 calories a day. Some of you may feel that you need to add in a few more, and I recommend that you work the numbers as I outlined in the preceding component. But, I would not increase to more than 1,500 calories for women or 1,800 calories for men until your body weight is where you want it to be and your energy trajectory is moving up. Even when both of those events occur, you always want to be monitoring your calories and never go back to your energy-destructive ways.

ALWAYS HAVE BALSAMIC VINEGAR OR FRESH LEMON OR LIME NEARBY

I am urging you to consume lots of fruits, vegetables, and lean protein, and nothing enhances the flavor in these foods more than balsamic vinegar or fresh lemon or lime. I

> ### A Word from Our Testers
> "During my 7 days, I was at a seminar and didn't have much time to prepare meals. The alternative—finding a steak house and having fish and a wedge lettuce salad with dressing on the side—worked great."
> *—Marsha M., age 56*

use balsamic vinegar on my grilled chicken, love it on salad or cut-up veggies, and truly use fresh lemon and lime the way most people use salt. Both lemon and lime up the taste, even of fruit, veggies, and almost all proteins. I keep them in my refrigerator at home and at my office and go through at least a dozen a week. Try it. And note, in the next component, Drink to Surge, you should add fresh lemon or lime to your water. It turns plain old water into something with a little more kick.

PREPARE GOOD-SMELLING FOODS

A recent study by the Smell & Taste Treatment and Research Foundation in Chicago proved that good-smelling foods translate directly into weight loss. They found that "smells are perceived as tastes, so they increase sensory satiety, making you feel full faster."[18] The study also showed that just slowing down and focusing on the smell of the food that you are eating works, but it never hurts to toss an apple in the microwave after you have stabbed it a few times. Ditto for a sweet potato or yam.

FOODS YOU SHOULD CONSUME SPARINGLY

OLIVE OIL

The media continually sing the praises of olive oil as if it can *only* be a plus for your body weight, health, and energy. I must respectfully disagree. Because olive oil is a plant-based monounsaturated fat, it *is* healthier than saturated or trans fats, such as those found in red meat, butter, and margarine, which clump up in the body and lead to hardening of the arteries, stroke, and heart disease. (You can tell the difference easily: Unsaturated fats are usually liquid at room temperature, while saturated and trans fats are solid at room temperature.) Unsaturated fats don't do this to the body, but olive oil is still 120 calories a tablespoon and 100 percent fat. You will soon understand how damaging it is to your energy to overeat. Dousing your salad, fish, vegetables, and bread in olive oil is *not* something I want you to do with any frequency.

If you would like to add a tablespoon or two to your favorite low-calorie dish, I say fine, but please, be sure to count those additional calories. *Do not* believe that olive oil possesses yet another "Get Out of Jail Free" card. I have purposely avoided it in the 7-Day Eating Surge because we are limiting calories this critical week.

Also note one of my favorite Karasisms:

Shine and glimmer won't make you slimmer.

If your grilled fish and veggies are shining back at you, then you must assume that they have been prepared with a great deal of oil and do not fall into the "energy-propelling, calorie-reducing" category.

SALAD DRESSING

We are consuming a staggering amount of calories in salad dressing. A while back, *Good Morning America* did a segment on dressing and determined that the average ladle of dressing used at a restaurant or salad bar contained approximately 450 calories. Yikes!

Don't be duped by supposed "light" dressings. Although they may possess less fat per serving, many of them are just as high in calories as the real thing.

At home, I recommend that you add very little low-calorie dressing to your salad and place it in either a spinner or a sealed Tupperware container and spin, spin, spin or shake, shake, shake. That way, the dressing is evenly disbursed on all the vegetables.

In a restaurant, *always* have the salad dressing served on the side; ideally, just ask for balsamic vinegar or fresh lemon or lime, as I previously urged you to do.

AVOCADO

Similar to olive oil, avocado possesses all the right, good fat, as opposed to the saturated fat previously described in the olive oil section. But it is also highly caloric; one medium-size avocado contains approximately 276 calories. That may not sound like much, but once you take the pit out and peel it, there really isn't that much avocado for that amount of calories. Avocado should be sprinkled on a salad or smeared on a turkey or chicken sandwich. Later in the book, you will learn that guacamole, whose base ingredient is avocado, is extremely high in calories and should be eaten very sparingly and not on the deep-fried chips presented at Mexican restaurants.

LEGUMES

All beans are a terrific source of protein, but they do add up in calories very quickly. A can of garbanzo beans, which my kids and I eat all the time (once we rinse them–virtually anything in a can is high in sodium and should be rinsed before eating), is a total of 350 calories. That, in itself, is not so bad, but you can overdo it with beans if you are not careful. Ditto with lentils. They are a great source of protein as well, especially for those who choose to eat a vegetarian diet, but they also add up in calories really fast.

As you will soon see in the eating plan, nuts, especially almonds and walnuts, are superfoods that possess just the right amount of protein, fat, and fiber. Purdue University researchers asked a group of women to add 334 calories of nuts each day, and the women did not gain any weight for the 10-week study period. The researchers concluded that the fiber in nuts might prevent your body from absorbing fat. Others believe that the fiber, protein, and fat make you feel full longer (I know it works for me), and nuts may even slightly increase calorie burning.[19]

But many people simply consume too, too many nuts. A small handful (which is probably what the 334 calories was) goes a long way. I am big on the benefits of nuts; just be careful of your portions! If you are looking to have a 100-calorie snack consisting of nuts, you may consume:

- 4 Brazil nuts
- 6 macadamia nuts
- 8 walnuts
- 10 pecans
- 11 hazelnuts
- 14 almonds
- 17 peanuts
- 25 pistachios

A Word from Our Testers

"I find around 3:30 to 6 p.m. the hardest time of the day (I feel a bit foggy then), but that snack does help. I am surprised at how well only 12 almonds can hold me over!"

—Andrew M., age 41

BEHAVIORS YOU SHOULD AVOID

SKIPPING BREAKFAST

Your mother was right; breakfast is the most important meal of the day. From a weight loss standpoint, research from the University of Massachusetts School of Medicine showed that "people who regularly skipped breakfast were a whopping 450 percent more likely to be overweight or obese than regular breakfast eaters."[20] Skipping breakfast can also lead to a 5 to 10 percent decrease, or slowing, of your basal metabolic rate, which is the amount of calories your body requires on a daily basis to stay alive. Your basal metabolic rate (BMR) is made up of the energy (calories) it takes for vital organs, such as the brain, lungs, heart, kidneys, liver, muscles, and skin, to name a few, to function.

Note: One of the most effective ways to increase BMR is to increase your lean muscle tissue–much more on that fact in Component 4, Exercise to Surge.

You're frequently going to hear me say that the human body is very, very smart. The reason your metabolism goes down when you skip breakfast is that by not eating in the morning, you are telling your brain that there is no readily available food source. Your brain thinks that you are stranded on a deserted island, therefore your metabolism must slow down to keep you alive longer. To effectively slow down, the body cannibalizes its most metabolically active tissue–precious muscle.

Never, ever do anything that breaks down your lean muscle tissue. Maintaining and increasing your lean muscle tissue causes your body to burn more calories, even at rest, which is essential to opulent energy. Please remember:

Metabolism Up = Energy Up

A substantial body of research also points to the fact that individuals who skip breakfast experience diminished energy and also a decreased ability to concentrate. If you can believe it, in the United States:

- One in eight children skip breakfast
- 15 percent of all teens skip breakfast
- One-third of all adults skip breakfast[21]

These are serious numbers. Every morning your blood sugar plummets due to the overnight fast, which will kill both concentration and energy because your brain can't store sugar (glucose) like the rest of the body and needs this glucose to function optimally. Skipping breakfast also causes you to "miss out on vital nutrients that promote peak cognition throughout the day," according to Katherine Tucker, PhD, professor of nutrition at Tufts University.[22]

Note: Most breakfast skippers are ravenous later in the morning. So what do they do? Choose quick, sugary, processed carbohydrates that further weaken their already impaired energy. That's the energy death spiral in action.

WAITING TOO LONG BETWEEN MEALS OR SNACKS

I know that I can't go longer than 4 hours–max–or my energy plummets. The reason this happens is that waiting too long in between meals or snacks causes blood sugar to drop, just as it does during sleep. You simply must keep blood sugar levels consistent, and that comes from eating the right foods every 3 to 4 hours.

Plus, eating enhances your metabolism (remember the saying I just introduced to you?), because digestion accounts for approximately 10 percent of your BMR.

And finally, when you skip meals or wait too long from one meal to the next, what do you generally do? Binge. Nothing zaps energy like a big splurge on unhealthy foods. . . . Thanksgiving ring a bell? I think you get the point.

DRIVING ON THE "SUGAR HIGHWAY"

Eating the "All White Diet" (white pasta, bread, rice, cookies, cake, cupcakes, muffins, etc.) and sugar is deadly to your health, your weight, and your energy.

Here's what happens when you eat white: You get up first thing in the morning and eat (that's good) a white bagel (oops, that's bad). That simple, white carbohydrate very quickly turns to sugar (glucose) in your bloodstream. It has what I refer to as a "very quick empty," which means little time in the stomach and direct dumping of sugar (glucose) into the bloodstream.

As a result of consuming that white bagel, you have a major league sugar party going on in your bloodstream. Now, the very smart human body says, "We have to get rid of all this sugar" and signals the pancreas to produce the hormone insulin. Think of insulin as the drawbridge to get the sugar into the castle (your cells and more). Without insulin, the sugar runs amok in your bloodstream (that's diabetes), causing damage to your eyesight, kidneys, heart, circulatory system . . . you name it. Raging blood sugar is a killer to your health *and* to your energy.

With excessive blood sugar, the pancreas steps up to the plate–big time–and releases an excessive amount of insulin. As a result, the sugar is quickly deposited into your cells, hopefully to be used for fuel, but more often than not, to be stored as body fat.

Then guess what happens? Your blood sugar is *so* low that you crash and burn with fatigue and brain fog, just like when you skip meals. What do you think most people do to get their blood sugar back up? They reach for another white edible that quickly turns to sugar that sends them cruising on that disastrous "Sugar Highway." Did you ever wonder why those muffins, cookies, candies, and brownies had such appeal at 10:00 a.m. *and* again at 4:00 p.m.?

In addition, higher insulin levels cause weight gain, inhibit the release of growth hormones, and suppress the immune system, which represent "The Bomb" when it comes to your energy.

We are facing an overwhelming diabetes epidemic in this country. Frequently, this is a result of excess body weight and excessive consumption of these damaging simple carbohydrates. When you continually panic the pancreas to pump out insulin in alarming quantities, the system ultimately breaks down and your cells actually become "insulin resistant," which means that even in the presence of insulin, the sugar continues to run rampant in your bloodstream and is not absorbed by your cells. That's the first step toward diabetes. You can control and avoid this situation simply by making smarter food choices.

During the next 7 days (and hopefully your lifetime), completely shun "The White." I mean it. It's not as difficult as you think, and the immediate energy fix is compelling.

CONSUMING TOO MANY CALORIES

According to the Centers for Disease Control and Prevention, women are consuming 22 percent more calories each day than they did in 1971. That fact alone may be the reason why women in their forties are 25 pounds heavier than they were in 1960, and that's for women in their forties. Most women experience their most significant weight gain as they approach menopause and that generally happens in the later forties to early fifties.[23]

This increased caloric intake is staggering in the long run, and it leads to substantial weight gain and profound smack to your energy.

With the recent restaurant trend toward gargantuan servings, we have lost all touch with reality when it comes to sensible portions. In the box below, New York University research lays out how our "average" portions of certain foods have skyrocketed in size and calories compared to the USDA recommendations:[24]

Food	20 years ago	Today
Cheeseburger	330 calories	590 calories
French fries	210 calories	610 calories
Blueberry muffin	210 calories	500 calories
Cookies		Now up 700 percent in size
Pasta portions		Now up 480 percent in size
Muffins		Now up 333 percent in size
Steaks		Now up 224 percent in size
Bagels		Now up 195 percent in size

These are very scary numbers that won't change unless we make conscientious choices when ordering in restaurants and buying food.

OVEREATING ON THE WEEKENDS

I have already mentioned the dangers associated with excessive weekend eating. I have noticed this for years with my clients in Chicago and New York, and now some new research concurs. According to a study in the journal *Obesity*, participants were broken up into the following two groups:

- One on a calorie-restricted (CR) diet
- One that exercised daily (ED)

The researchers found that the CR group stopped losing weight on the weekends and that the ED group gained weight from splurging on the weekends.[25]

Think about your eating as you would your money. If you save all week, then blow it on the weekend, you end up at ground zero on Monday or maybe even in the hole (which, in this instance, is weight *gain*). To keep this from happening, seriously consider my previous recommendations regarding keeping a food diary, weighing yourself frequently, and wearing jeans on the weekends. Trust me, that's a winning (as in losing) combination.

EATING CAESAR SALAD

I can't tell you how damaging this salad, if you can even call it a salad, is to your energy boost. Caesar salad is a deadly combination of oil, cheese, egg, and fried croutons. Now, on their own, a little oil, as I earlier explained, cheese, and egg is fine, but when blended together on your innocent, low-calorie, energy-producing romaine lettuce, these harmless leaves quickly turn from Dr. Jekyll into Mr. Hyde. Drop the croutons on top and you are headed to about a 750-plus calorie disaster. Stop it. The most often eaten salad in the United States is the Caesar, and look at the obesity mess we have gotten ourselves into. Again, Caesar must be stopped!

SADDLING UP TO FAST FOOD

I realize this is somewhat obvious, because the majority of the items you will find in fast-food establishments are not, in general, energy producing as they are *loaded* in calories. A study reported in the *Annals of Internal Medicine* showed that even people at a healthier weight misjudged the calories in larger fast-food meals by a whopping 22.6 to 38 percent.[26] Plus, the journal *Gut* chronicled a Swedish study that asked 18 lean, healthy medical students to adopt a sedentary lifestyle and eat two fast-food meals a day for 1 month. On average, the students gained 14.1 pounds, 2.6 inches to their waist, and 3.7 percent body fat.[27]

I almost placed this in the "consume sparingly" category because there *are* some options at almost every fast-food restaurant that could be considered energy enhancing, and they include:

McDonald's	Calories	Fat	Sodium
Grilled Chicken Classic Sandwich	420	10g	1,190 mg
without mayo	*370*	*4.5 g*	*1,110 mg*
without mayo and half bun	*250*	*2.75 g*	*910 mg*
Southwest Grilled Chicken Salad (no dressing)	320	9 g	960 mg
with Newman's Own Southwest Dressing	*420*	*15 g*	*1,300 mg*
with Newman's Own Low-Fat Balsamic Dressing	*360*	*12 g*	*1,690 mg*
Burger King	**Calories**	**Fat**	**Sodium**
TENDERGRILL Chicken Sandwich	510	19 g	1,180 mg
without mayo	*400*	*7 g*	*1,090 mg*
without mayo and half bun	*275*	*5.25 g*	*845 mg*
TENDERGRILL Garden Salad (no dressing)	240	9 g	720 mg
with Ken's Light Italian Dressing	*360*	*20 g*	*1,160 mg*
with Ken's Fat-Free Ranch Dressing	*290*	*9 g*	*1,460 mg*
Wendy's	**Calories**	**Fat**	**Sodium**
Grilled Chicken Go Wrap	260	11 g	760 mg
substitute regular mustard for the honey mustard	*230*	*8 g*	*760 mg*
*Ultimate Chicken Grill with cheese	380	12 g	1,280 mg
*Ultimate Chicken Grill without cheese	320	7 g	950 mg
substitute regular mustard for the honey mustard	*280*	*4 g*	*940 mg*
Salads here have between 400 and 600 calories unless you substitute everything on the salad. The above are better selections.			
Subway	**Calories**	**Fat**	**Sodium**
6" Turkey Breast Sandwich on Whole Wheat	280	4.5 g	1,000 mg
Oven Roasted Chicken Salad (no dressing)	140	2.5 g	400 mg
with Fat-Free Italian Dressing	*175*	*2.5 g*	*1,120 mg*
Quizno's	**Calories**	**Fat**	**Sodium**
Small Tuscan Turkey on Rosemary Parmesan	420	17.5 g	1,195 mg
without cheese and dressing	*280*	*4.5 g*	*1,070 mg*
Small Honey Bourbon Chicken Sandwich	320	4.5 g	900 mg

**My Choice—almost double the protein*

I am going to ask you to change many behaviors this coming week. (If you'd like a sneak peek, you'll find the 7-day eating plan laid out in Part II.) One of the simplest things you can do is adjust what you put into your mouth. This isn't a function of time or money; it's simply a decision by you to make better choices. It starts with a trip to the grocery store or just reaching for the energy-lifting food you keep buying with good intentions, but often neglect. No one forces you to eat certain foods. You make that decision. The effects that these foods and behaviors will have on your energy are profound and immediate. Talk about instant gratification!

COMPONENT 3

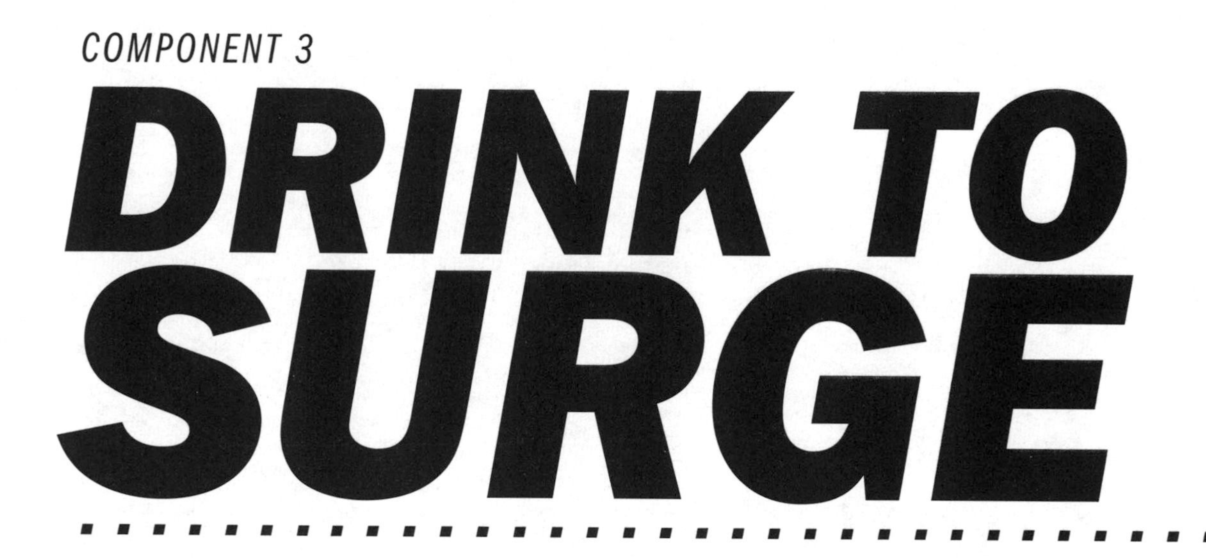

DRINK TO SURGE

Americans are drinking way too much of the wrong liquids and not enough of the right ones. They think that if it's liquid, it doesn't count, and they routinely guzzle orange juice and soda and "designer" coffees (aka milkshakes) or even load *regular* old coffee and tea with tons of cream and sugar. According to a 2007 analysis of government data on U.S. beverage trends, Americans are drinking one-quarter of their average daily caloric intake.[1] Did you have any idea that 25 percent of your caloric intake was coming from something that you never had to chew?

Here is a study that I truly want you to read over and over again–Purdue University researchers took 120 people, half lean and half obese, and had them either drink or eat foods with similar properties and calories: watermelon juice versus watermelon with the same amount of carbohydrates, coconut milk and coconut meat with the same amount of fat, milk and cheese with the same amount of protein, etc. In addition to these test meals, the individuals could eat whatever they wanted for the rest of the day. The results showed that total caloric intake was 12 to 19 percent *higher* when the participants consumed the liquid calories rather than the solid food, and they theorized that liquid calories simply don't tip the satiety mechanism the way solid food does. Translation–STOP drinking your calories.[2]

Remember my discussion in the preceding chapter about the insulin response to foods that quickly turn into sugar? The same applies to liquid calories. If you run out the door in the morning with juice in hand, you have started your day on the "Sugar Highway." Naturally, you then stop for some coffee (more often than not, laden with additional calories), which frequently includes the caffeine hit, which I refer to as the one-two punch of "chemical" energy. Congratulations: You are now plummeting down the energy death spiral.

Liquids you should drink more of

☐ Water

☐ Tea

☐ Soup*

☐ Wheatgrass juice

Liquids you should drink sparingly

☐ Coffee

☐ Milk

☐ Protein drinks/shakes

- ☐ Alcohol, including wine, beer, and hard liquor
- ☐ Soup*

Liquids you should avoid

- ☐ Diet soda
- ☐ Regular soda
- ☐ Juice
- ☐ Sports drinks
- ☐ Energy drinks
- ☐ Soup*

*I realize that soup is showing up on all three lists, which must seem confusing, but you will soon understand why.

LIQUIDS YOU SHOULD DRINK MORE OF

WATER

Water is the "gold standard" when it comes to optimizing energy, because the human body is made up of 60 to 75 percent water, and the brain 85 percent water! When dehydrated, a typical state for many people, the body lacks balance and fatigues readily. I know that when I am dehydrated, I feel like I am getting the flu. As I said in the introduction to this book, most people only drink water when they pop a pill for a headache: Chances are, that headache is most likely brought on by dehydration.

Many people are totally confused about water balance. When dehydrated, the very smart human body says, "There isn't a readily available source of water," just as it does when we skip meals. When in distress, the body's survival mechanism kicks in and says, "Hey, we need to hold on to all the water because there's none coming in" and retains water to survive, mostly in the wrong places: stomach, chin, cheeks, hands, feet, and thighs–you know, water bloat. You don't want this to happen. Did you know that humans can survive weeks without food but very few days (as in two, max three) without water? Water is that essential.

Many women say to me, "Jim, I just can't drink water because I'm already bloated." I explain the bloat is from dehydration. Once you drink water, the opposite signal is sent to the body and it releases the reserves. You lean out *and* feel a significant energy spurt.

The $64,000 question is "How much water do we really need daily?" We regularly hear eight, 8-ounce glasses of water a day (64 ounces), while others claim we should consume half our body weight in ounces.

I disagree with the experts who claim we really don't need that much water, because they don't take into account the following issues:

- Body weight–The more you weigh, the more water you need. I hope that makes sense.
- Exercise–Perspiration is your body's cooling mechanism and requires more water. The more you work out, the more water you require.
- Climate–I just got back from three days in the desert in Las Vegas and was drinking water like a madman because of the dryness. Ditto in cold climates where we are accosted by forced, dry air in our homes, offices, stores, and restaurants, which is why humidifiers EVERYWHERE, at that time of year, are a must.
- Medication–Certain medications rob the body of water.
- Sodium–Salt and the sodium content in certain foods (canned goods and just about everything you eat out) rob your body of water. Did you know that you should only consume 2,300 milligrams of sodium a day (that's just a teaspoon of salt) and that daily salt consumption has gone from 2,300 milligrams in the 1970s to 3,300 milligrams today? That's a big jump and a major energy hit.
- Alcohol–I will soon talk about this in more detail, but when you drink alcohol, it depletes your body of water.
- Cabin pressure–Do you know the difference in humidity between cabin pressure and the Sahara Desert? Zip, zero, nada. Flying is brutal on water balance and energy, which is why it is essential to pound down the water when flying.

Do you want more reasons to hit the H_2O?

- A study reported by the University of North Carolina at Chapel Hill proved that those who drink water regularly consume about 200 fewer calories a day than those who only consume tea, coffee, or soda. Drink more water every day and that will lead to losing close to 21 pounds a year. A clear energy upper.[3]

- A spanking new study in the *Journal of Applied Physiology* showed that dehydration keeps your body from losing fat and gaining strength after resistance exercise because it increases stress hormones (body fat up, muscle down), lessens testosterone production (body fat up, muscle down), and alters carbohydrate and fat metabolism (you guessed it, body fat up, muscle down).[4]
- German researchers have found that water fuels your ability to burn fat for fuel, which is clearly highly desirable. For approximately 90 minutes after drinking chilled water (remember in the introduction I told you to go get a big glass of cold, sparkling water?), participants showed that their metabolism increased by 24 percent (approximately 50 calories), which researchers believe was partially due to the energy your body expends to warm up the water while digesting. You will lose 5 additional pounds each year just by following the cold-water prescription (approximately 48 ounces) because an increase in metabolism, with all other variables remaining constant, will result in weight loss.[5, 6]
- Chewing ice increases metabolism. Although it may be rough on your teeth, chewing the ice in your drinks may burn an additional 70 extra calories a day.[7]
- Most people misinterpret thirst as hunger. By drinking a big glass of cold water instead of reaching for something to eat, you will find your energy increases while your waist decreases.

Bottom line–water is *always* energy positive and, with the exception of a New York City marathon runner (FYI–marathons should be abolished; more on that later) who consumed gallons upon gallons of water and died, I have never heard of illness or harm befalling anyone drinking a lot of water. If you plan on drinking 5 to 6 gallons, that is a whole other story and is *not* my recommendation.

For the record, I don't care whether your preference is tap, bottled, spring, or still water; just make sure it doesn't contain hidden calories. If you like sparkling water (I do), you may get a double bang for your buck. A new study in the *British Journal of Nutrition* found that drinking sparkling water actually increases satiety (remember that word from our discussion of liquid versus solid calories) and, therefore, decreases the amount of calories consumed. I'd give that a try.[8]

I'm also a fan of flavored water. Just be careful to read the label and choose a brand that's lower in calories. Try it if you aren't a big water fan; my kids drink it and love it.

And finally, *all* liquids, including caffeinated and decaffeinated coffee, tea, soda (regular and diet), juice, and even low-sodium soup, do count toward your water intake. In the past, researchers said that caffeinated drinks did not count because they have a diuretic effect, but they have since changed their position. Foods with a high water content, such as fruits and vegetables, also count.

TEA

Did you know that tea is the second most commonly consumed liquid (water being #1) in the world? Drinking tea may possibly be one of the simplest ways to bring forth heightened energy *and* health, because it has been shown to:

- **Help keep lost weight off.** A Dutch study followed people who had successfully lost weight and found that those who drank green tea kept losing weight while those on the placebo regained as much as 40 percent of the lost weight.[9] A Taiwanese study over a 10-year period showed that drinking green, black, or oolong tea a few times a week resulted in 20 percent less body fat compared to the placebo beverage. They believe that certain tea extracts (called catechins, an antioxidant) increase metabolism (remember, Metabolism Up = Energy Up).[10] Some estimates put this boost to metabolism around 4 percent to as high as 12 percent.
- **Boost exercise performance.** Japanese researchers found that when mice were given green-tea extract their endurance improved twice as much as those given the placebo. The researchers believe that tea helps muscles "process lipids and use fatty acids as an energy source." Humans would need about 4 cups a day to duplicate the results.[11]
- **Build long, lean, calorie-burning muscles.** Brazilian scientists showed that consuming three cups of green tea a day helped muscles recover faster after intense strength training because the participants had fewer markers of cell damage.[12]
- **Boost your brain power.** According to John Foxe, PhD, professor of neuroscience, biology, and psychology at the City College of New York, an amino acid, theanine, present almost exclusively in black, green, and oolong tea, can produce "significant

improvements in tests for attention, and that activity in the cortical regions responsible for attention functions are enhanced. In just 20 minutes after consuming theanine, the blood concentrations increase and the brain's alpha waves are impacted."[13]

- **Reduce the risk of heart disease and high cholesterol.** Research shows that regular tea drinkers are 44 percent less likely to suffer a heart attack. For those who did suffer one, tea helped them recover faster.[14]
- **Prevent Parkinson's disease.** A new study followed 63,000 middle-aged and older people for 7 years and found that those who consumed 6 ounces of tea a day dramatically reduced their risk of this disease. The researchers said that caffeine was a factor, but that there had to be something else in the black tea that caused this reduction, because green tea had no positive effect.[15]

I am a huge tea drinker, mostly green, but with splashes of black and white. I believe it has made a significant difference in my body weight, health, and overall energy. Year-round, I brew tea in my office (okay, I don't do it, my assistant does . . . didn't want to lie!), then place it in a big container in the refrigerator and drink it cold, over ice. I recommend that you drink three cups of tea a day, but feel free to consume more if you stay within the 300-milligram caffeine limit. I also strongly urge you to drink tea with as little sweetener (if any) as possible.

SOUP

I realize that it must be confusing to see soup in all three categories. When you read this entire chapter, you will understand why. In general, most soup is *totally* energy negative, but there are two soups that are clearly energy positive and they are:

- **Homemade soup prepared with very, very little sodium.** If you are making soup from scratch and are using low-sodium stock sparingly and preparing a big pot of vegetable soup with water, seasoning, and possibly some added protein, I say great. If you are upping the sodium count with certain ingredients, such as soy sauce, bouillon, or plain old salt, then you must stop consuming this energy-depleting concoction.
- **Bieler's Broth.** Renowned physician and author Dr. Henry Bieler was ahead of his time back in the 1960s, when he emphasized diet and lifestyle for disease prevention. He identified that in the human body, blood and saliva shift in pH balance from

alkaline (good) to acidic (bad). If the body is too acidic, it will withdraw alkaline minerals from bones, soft tissue, body fluids, and saliva. An acidic body state is a breeding ground for degenerative disease and frequently results from consuming

Heartland Stew

In my second book, *Flip the Switch*, I included a recipe for Heartland Stew, which is a fantastic vegetable stew with flavor, fiber, and very, very few calories. It's a Karas staple in my house. Check it out.

HEARTLAND STEW

Number of servings: 8

Calories per serving: 185

Preparation time: 2 hours

2 quarts vegetable stock

2 medium potatoes, cut into large chunks (I like them unpeeled, but you can peel if you like)

1 cup cooked pinto or kidney beans (if you use canned, then rinse them well)

2 medium tomatoes, diced into ½-inch chunks

½ pound carrots, peeled and cut into large chunks

2 parsnips, diced into ½-inch chunks (optional)

1 medium yellow onion, cut into ½-inch chunks

2 cups green cabbage, cut into large chunks and leaves separated

1 green bell pepper, cut into large pieces

2 6-ounce cans tomato paste

1½ teaspoons sage

1 bunch green onions, chopped (white and green parts)

salt and pepper to taste

Place all ingredients, except the green onions and salt and pepper, into a large stockpot. Bring to a boil and simmer for 1 to 1½ hours, or until the desired thickness is reached. Add the chopped green onions. Season to taste and serve.

BIELER'S BROTH

A Potent, Energy-Expanding Elixir

3 bunches of parsley, rinsed very well and stems cut off

1½ pounds green beans, ends cut off

2½ pounds zucchini, ends cut off and sliced into chunks

Place the parsley, green beans, and zucchini in a big pot, then add enough water to cover the vegetables by 1 inch. Bring to a boil, cover, and simmer for 30 minutes, until a fork easily pierces the zucchini. Let cool, then puree in batches in a blender or food processor, adding in some of the vitamin-rich water. The consistency should resemble pea soup.

This recipe should make approximately 21 cups, or enough for all 7 days of the Surge. Ideally, keep it in a glass container, cutting back on the plastic, which is not good for your health or the environment.

NOTE: Do not add any salt, seasoning, or anything else to this sacred, medicinal potion.

sugar and simple carbohydrates and also from experiencing excessive stress. Bieler's Broth supplies the basic building blocks (precious minerals–calcium, magnesium, chlorophyll, natural sodium, and potassium) for an ideal alkaline body. That is why you will be consuming this broth on a daily basis.

WHEATGRASS JUICE

If you really want to go the extra mile, drink wheatgrass juice. There has been considerable attention paid to the vast benefits of wheatgrass. With regard to the energy surge, wheatgrass:

- **Stimulates metabolism**–remember, Metabolism Up = Energy Up.
- **Enhances mental concentration,** which enables you to get more done in a given period of time.
- **Provides powerful antioxidants,** which promote health and reduce the damaging effects of aging.

- **Balances blood sugar and blood pressure.**
- **Regenerates the liver,** your primary detoxification organ.
- **Alkalinizes the body** (reread the section on Bieler's Broth if you forgot how important this is).

Therefore, on a daily basis, you might consume one shot of wheatgrass juice each day. The juice is available at Jamba Juice, Whole Foods, and other health food stores. You can also prepare it at home by purchasing fresh wheatgrass and juicing it; by purchasing dry wheatgrass under the labels Green Magma, Greens+, and Kyo-Green; or by purchasing freeze-dried wheatgrass, which you add to water. Just know that the juice has to be consumed within 5 minutes after preparation or it starts to lose some of its most beneficial properties.

For the record, wheatgrass has only 5 calories per ounce.

LIQUIDS YOU SHOULD DRINK SPARINGLY

COFFEE

Roughly 54 percent of Americans 18 and older drink coffee daily, and 30 percent consume it occasionally.[16] There has been considerable debate over whether coffee is energy positive or energy negative, and whether it prevents disease or promotes it. It also depends on what you define as "coffee" and whether it is caffeinated, decaffeinated, or liquid dessert (did anyone say Frappuccino?). Caffeine levels also vary tremendously, from 330 milligrams at Starbucks to 145 milligrams at Dunkin' Donuts for the same size cup.

The pros and cons that I am going to debate pertain to coffee–plain old coffee–not a calorie-laden milkshake masquerading as coffee.

Here are the benefits:

- **Increased alertness.** According to one research study conducted by the University of Oklahoma, caffeinated coffee makes you feel sharper. There is a compound called adenosine, which builds up in the body throughout the day and causes you to slow down and become sleepy. Adenosine is frequently referred to as "Nature's Chill Pill." When adenosine and caffeine compete for the same receptors, caffeine wins and stimulates your central nervous system and brain. BAM! You feel alert. The recommended dosage is generally 100 to 200 milligrams of caffeine per cup, but it will need to be increased as you become more accustomed to the jolt.[17] I like that for a quick hit of energy, when needed, but it does fall under the heading of "chemical" energy and should be used sparingly.

Note: This increased alertness comes with a price, because it causes production of the stress hormones adrenaline and cortisol (much more on them in Component 8). Some people, after the initial "rush," which lasts about 45 minutes for a 100 milligram cup, may then "crash." This may necessitate *more* coffee.[18] Don't do that; cut back and feel your energy levels balance out and use caffeinated coffee only when necessary.

- **Slower cellular damage.** Americans get the majority of their antioxidants from coffee. This is unfortunately the case; they should be getting the majority of their antioxidants from fruits and vegetables instead. Antioxidants are molecules that slow or prevent cellular damage caused by free radicals. Free radicals are incomplete and unstable oxygen molecules that rob and destroy healthy cells. Antioxidants run interference and stop this damaging, energy-robbing process. If you can believe it, coffee has four times the antioxidants of green tea. Slowing cellular damage also reduces the risk of certain diseases and makes you feel young.
- **Added calorie burn.** Because caffeinated coffee stimulates the central nervous system (brain and spinal cord), it boosts your metabolism anywhere from 5 to 8 percent, which translates into approximately 98 to 174 additional calories burned a day. That really adds up when it comes to weight loss and energy.[19]
- **Diminished risk of cardiovascular disease.** A study published in the *Annals of Internal Medicine* looked at 41,736 men and 86,216 women for 18 and 24 years, respectively. They found that as coffee consumption increased, the risk of death from cardiovascular disease decreased. This occurred while the participants were drinking both caffeinated and decaffeinated coffee, so the researchers theorize that it's not the caffeine but other compounds in coffee that provide the benefit.[20]

  In another 2006 study, Norwegian researchers discovered that by drinking one to three cups of coffee each day, older women reduced their risk of cardiovascular disease by 24 percent.[21] This is significant given the fact that women now outnumber men in the yearly death toll from heart disease.

- **Reduced risk of type 2 diabetes.** Since 2002, more than 20 case studies have shown that drinking either caffeinated or decaffeinated coffee reduces the risk of this disease. According to the American Diabetic Association, 23.6 million adults and children (8 percent of our population) currently have diabetes and 5.7 million of those 23.6 million do NOT know they have the disease. And the following statistic is staggering. According to the CDC's Capital Morbidity and Mortality Weekly Report, 4 percent of Americans report being diagnosed as "prediabetic."[22] Unfortunately, one-quarter of Americans actually have prediabetes and don't even know it. My son Evan was born in 2000, and researchers believe that one-third of all children born that year will ultimately become diabetic. As for prevention, researchers believe that it's not just the caffeine in coffee but other compounds as well that help reduce the risk. In 2005, Harvard researchers determined that men and women will cut their risk of developing diabetes by 50 percent and 30 percent, respectively, by drinking six cups of caffeinated coffee a day. How this is not plastered on the cover of every paper is mind-boggling to me.[23]

  Another researcher theorizes that a compound in coffee, chlorogenic acid, delays sugar (glucose) from being absorbed in the intestines, which would help reduce the spikes in blood sugar that I wrote about in Component 2. Reducing blood sugar spikes will help discourage diabetes *and* enhance energy.
- **Less risk of liver and colon cancers.** Research from the National Cancer Center in Tokyo found that drinking caffeinated coffee reduced the risk of liver cancer, and the more participants drank, the more the risk diminished.[24] That same study also showed that regular coffee consumption lowered a woman's risk of colon cancer by 50 percent. A German study confirmed these findings; those researchers identified a powerful antioxidant compound that boosts the "activity of phase II enzymes, which are thought to protect against colon cancer."[25]
- **Lower risk of Parkinson's disease.** One and a half million Americans suffer from Parkinson's (most visibly the actor Michael J. Fox), and drinking 100 to 200 milligrams of caffeinated coffee a day can reduce your risk by 30 percent. Harvard researchers claim that drinking up to four cups a day will cut your risk in half.[26] Caffeine stimulates the release of dopamine, a brain chemical that is responsible for increased alertness, enhanced pleasure, and even superior problem solving. Dopa-

mine levels diminish with Parkinson's disease, but the caffeine in coffee helps keep them active, which is why your risk lowers with each cup.

- **Prevention of gallstones.** The Nurses' Health Study showed that those who drank four cups of regular, caffeinated coffee had a significantly lower risk of developing gallstones than those who did not drink coffee. Those who drank five or more cups reduced their risk even further.[27]
- **Improved skin.** Want to feel more energized when you get up in the morning? How about seeing fewer wrinkles (that would work for me!)? A new study published in *Cancer Research* showed that "caffeine sloughs off the skin cells that become damaged by the sun." They go on to say that drinking three to five cups of coffee a day (though they don't give the exact milligrams of caffeine, nor do they say whether other caffeinated beverages also provide the same benefit) would do the job.[28]

The negative effects of drinking coffee include:

- **The "Caffeine Highway."** Similar to the way that processed carbs cause a spike in blood sugar, followed by a surge of insulin and then a "crash," coffee is a stimulant that fires up your adrenals and causes excessive adrenaline and cortisol to be pumped out, leaving you jittery and nervous. A full day on the "Caffeine Highway" is not energy positive.
- **Elevated inflammatory markers.** Two different studies showed that 200 milligrams of coffee raised homocysteine levels (an indicator of inflammation) and upped the risk of heart disease. While the research I cited shows coffee to reduce heart disease, this research contradicts it and says that coffee actually increases it.[29] I'm sure more research will come along in the very near future as the debate continues.
- **Fertility problems and birth defects.** Pregnant women should be very careful with coffee, because it has been associated with premature birth, birth defects, inability to conceive, low birth weight, and miscarriage. Guys aren't exempt, because coffee consumption has been linked to sluggish sperm.
- **Cancer.** Although coffee may help prevent some cancers, it may also aggravate others, such as stomach cancer and leukemia.
- **Sleep disruption.** As I mentioned earlier, caffeinated coffee blocks adenosine, the brain chemical (again, Nature's Chill Pill) that prepares the body for sleep. By blocking this

chemical, you'll feel perky, but if you drink coffee too late in the day, your sleep might be disrupted. As a general rule, you should stop drinking coffee by noon. If you can believe it, my 85-year-old grandmother (who has since passed) used to get up in the middle of the night and pump down six cups of percolated coffee (which is loaded with caffeine) and fall right back into blissful sleep, so it doesn't affect everyone the same way.

A Word from Our Testers

"I stopped drinking coffee a few months ago but I really improved my energy score when I started drinking more water and tea."

—Colleen M., age 39

Coffee can either be energy/health positive or negative. In general, stay under 300 milligrams of caffeine a day, and don't drink coffee after noon if you have sleeping issues. However, if you are at risk for heart disease, diabetes, liver and colon cancer, or Parkinson's disease, you may want to drink a little more. Weigh the pros and cons carefully, consult with your doctor as necessary, and decide what's the right amount of coffee for you.

MILK

I've already addressed the issue of calcium-rich dairy on page 14, but I specifically want to look at the benefits of milk postexercise.

A research study took 56 men, average age 22, who were new to weight training, and had them strength-train for 12 weeks. Postworkout, they were given nonfat milk, a soy-based drink, or a carbohydrate drink.

At the end of the 12 weeks, the results showed that:

- The milk drinkers gained 8.8 pounds of muscle and lost 2 pounds of body fat.
- The soy drinkers gained 6 pounds of muscle and barely lost any body fat.
- The carbohydrate drinkers gained 5.3 pounds of muscle and lost 1 pound of body fat.

The researchers speculate that the proteins in milk, such as whey and caseins, and the calcium may be responsible for the difference.[30]

And remember from the previous chapter that consuming high-protein, high-fat foods postexercise enhances the afterburn, so you might want to reach for 2 percent milk.

As with coffee, you need to determine the right amount of milk to consume on a daily basis, and you should take into consideration whether or not you exercised, how many calories you plan on consuming that day, etc. In general, keep your low-fat milk consumption to ½ to 1 cup per day. It would be ideal if you had your first ½ cup with cereal in the morning, then another ½ cup postexercise.

PROTEIN DRINKS/SHAKES

This is a difficult category, so I want to break it up between the drinks and shakes you personally make and those that are purchased.

If you don't know exactly what is in a shake when you purchase it, then avoid it. These drinks could easily contain 500+ calories and pounds of sugar. Unless you are using them as a major meal replacement or plowing the fields for 8 hours a day, I would avoid them.

If you're at home and you'd like to mix some 1 or 2 percent milk (not juice), fresh or frozen sugar-free berries, and protein powder in a portion-controlled manner, fine. But remember the words *portion-controlled*; if you just start dumping, odds are you are going to consume too many calories.

Note: I do like protein shakes, in a portion-controlled manner, as a postworkout snack; remember how important it is to eat the right foods immediately after your interval strength training.

During the first week, please stick with the meal plan provided. Protein shakes may be an option after the 7-Day Energy Surge, but do approach them cautiously and know every ingredient and the corresponding caloric value.

ALCOHOL, INCLUDING WINE, BEER, AND HARD LIQUOR

The research is pretty clear with regard to how much wine, beer, or hard liquor you should drink for your health.

Women may consume 13 to 15 grams of alcohol a day, which equals:

- **One 5-ounce glass of wine** (approximately 100 to 125 calories)
- **A 12-ounce bottle of beer** (and I hope it's "light," at between 65 and 90 calories, versus double or more than that for the real deal)
- **A 1.5-ounce shot of 80-proof liquor**

It might not be wise for women to drink every day because of the link between breast cancer and alcohol, but that is something for you to discuss with your doctor, at your physical, which you better have scheduled by now. For the record, having one or two drinks a day ups a woman's risk of breast cancer by 10 percent and three or more a day increases the risk by 30 percent.[31, 32]

Men can drink twice as much simply because they are bigger and can therefore metabolize more alcohol. Consuming moderate amounts of alcohol would be considered energy positive for most because of the health benefits. If it interferes with your sleep patterns, then I would avoid it.

Once you go above those maximums, however, you are clearly in energy-negative territory. Tell me, how did you feel the morning after a big night of eating and drinking? Probably not ready to scale Mt. Everest.

To prevent that, I want you to remember to *always* be a two-fisted drinker. What I mean by that is consume 2 ounces of water for every ounce of alcohol. Following that strategy will enable you to:

- **Drink less** because you will fill up with water.
- **Feel so much better** in the morning from hydration.
- **Look so much better.** As I mentioned earlier, when you are dehydrated, you puff up. You will counter that by drinking tons of water the night before and first thing in the morning.

Clearly, there are other components of too much drinking that are energy negative, such as car accidents, falls, disease, loose lips (which includes saying the wrong thing *and* kissing the wrong person) . . . I think you get the point.

To Drink or Not to Drink?

A recent study found that drinking more than one drink increased your risk of metabolic syndrome, especially for women; more than one drink raised women's risk by 60 percent.[33]

SOUP

Okay, I clearly love, love, love the Bieler's Broth (page 38) and the Heartland Stew (page 37) and anything you make at home with very low sodium and virtually no added fat. But I am also a fan of the no calorie, low sodium soups. If you look at the labels, you will see that they are far lower in sodium than their full-leaded counterparts, so for that reason, I do feel they can be consumed from time to time. If you *really* want to make me happy, then you would add some extra vegetables, lean protein, and water to the contents of the can.

LIQUIDS YOU SHOULD AVOID

DIET SODA

Okay, because I just told you I am a huge tea drinker, I want to come clean and tell you that I used to be an *enormous* consumer of Diet X. I easily pumped down 10+ cans a day. No, that is not a typo; I easily drank 10+ cans a day. *Chicago* magazine did an article called "A Day in the Life of Jim Karas," and I lied in the article and said that I had one can of Diet X with breakfast and another with lunch. My staff read it, looked at me, tilted their heads, and said, "Right! What about the other 100 ounces you guzzle down the rest of the day?" They called me out, and that was the catalyst for me to get off what I called "The Juice"; for the past three years, not a single drop has crossed my lips. I feel so much healthier and recall an immediate, positive shift in my energy.

Research in 2008 found that consuming just one can of diet soda a day increased the risk of metabolic syndrome by 34 percent. Even the lead researcher doesn't really understand why and wonders whether it is a chemical in the diet soda that is causing this reaction, or whether it is more about the behavior of people who drink it. Stay tuned, as I am sure more studies will follow.[34]

REGULAR SODA

Simply put, soda is a *disaster* for your energy, your health, your teeth, your body weight, and I could just go on and on and on. Regular soda is 12 calories an ounce. In the olden

Artificial Sweeteners

I am frequently asked, "What are the safest artificial sweeteners?" My answer—I don't know. Sure, the researchers say that they "appear" not to cause cancer, memory loss, or any of the other often discussed consequences of consuming too many artificial sweeteners (which may include growing a second head). A case study conducted at the University of California, San Diego, showed that consuming Splenda (sucralose) rather than sugar (sucrose) could lead people to crave *more* sweets rather than satisfy the sweet craving, which is what happened when participants consumed "the real thing."[35] I'm sure more research is on the horizon, but in general, I would strongly urge you to use any artificial sweetener sparingly, if at all, and don't shun good old-fashioned sugar or honey (more on honey in the sex component. HHHMMMM????), because they may actually be the best choice when used in a small, portion-controlled manner.

days, people drank those little 8-ounce bottles for a total of 96 calories, and some were even smaller. Today, we walk around with tubs filled with 20, 30, 40, or more ounces of soda for a grand total of 240, 360, 480, or more calories. Whenever I ride the subway in Chicago and New York, I almost always see overweight teens drinking vats of sugar-laden soda.

Harvard researcher David Ludwig, MD, PhD, found that the odds of a child becoming obese increased by 60 percent with each additional sugar-sweetened drink, which may mean soda or juice (just wait until you hear my opinion of juice!). That's a *huge* increase per serving and a reason to get all soda and juice out of the mouths of babes *and* children.

Ludwig also pointed out that it is not uncommon for teens to pump down 500 to 1,000 calories each and every day from a sugary drink. That will destroy a teen's energy and send him or her on an energy roller coaster all day and into the night.[36]

Cutting back on regular soda consumption is not enough. I say totally eliminate it. Period. The moment you do, you will feel such a huge difference in your energy. You will be off the sugar and caffeine highways and on your way to a lower body weight. That's a great energy-positive decision.

JUICE

Okay, you think I was tough on regular soda? Fasten your seat belt: Juice is even worse. Yes, you read that correctly; juice is a disaster when it comes to energy. Did you know that juice has even *more* calories than soda?

A while back, the Chicago public schools removed soda from vending machines and substituted juice. Oh, great: Soda has 12 calories an ounce and juice has 15. We just gave our kids 25 percent more liquid calories. Not a solution, if you ask me.

And don't start with the, "What if it's freshly squeezed?" You are far better off eating the orange, pulp, fiber, and all.

I fly a lot in what my kids call "The Big Seat," and now, on many flights, juice and water are offered before takeoff. I play a little game with myself and guess, in advance, who will drink the juice and who will drink the water. I'm at about a 97 percent accuracy rating because I can instantly tell, just by their appearance, which drink people will choose.

Just stop drinking juice! A few times in this book I am going to get emphatic, and this is one of those times. It's a disaster for your body and energy all around.

SPORTS DRINKS

As I lecture all over the world on enhancing energy, optimizing body weight, and stalling if not reversing the aging process, I am almost always asked, "Are sports drinks okay?" My answer: "If you are on the 21st mile of a marathon (which I hope you never, ever run, because marathons are brutal on your body and your energy and, as I earlier stated, should be abolished) or in the fifth set against Roger Federer at Wimbledon (if you should be so lucky), fine." If you are not in either of those two situations, then get rid of the sports drinks. It is a marketing sham and the whole "you need to replace your electrolytes when exercising" argument doesn't stand up in case studies. Plus, no one needs the extra calories that they provide. Water does the trick. Again, water does the trick.

ENERGY DRINKS

Energy drinks, such as Red Bull and Monster drinks, are astonishingly popular because they are readily available, can be mixed with alcohol for a caffeine *and* alcohol bump, and appeal to people of all ages. I know a number of celebrities and CEOs in their sixties and seventies who live on these drinks for the "chemical energy" hit.

Eight ounces of Red Bull contains 110 calories and 80 milligrams of caffeine; Monster drinks possess the same caffeine and only 100 calories per serving. My vote is to put regular soda, juice, and energy drinks in the same category. Get rid of them. I would much rather see you drink some coffee or tea in the morning if you feel you need the caffeine lift, because they also contain powerful antioxidants.

SOUP—AGAIN!

Soup in a restaurant, full-sodium can, salad bar, or deli is a *disaster* when it comes to your energy. Are any of you *Seinfeld* fans? I am a huge one. Do you remember the Soup Nazi? Are you ready for this?

"No Soup for You!"

He was absolutely right, and if you want to optimize energy, you will never have another drop of this category of soup cross your lips, because it is an amalgam of:

- **Sodium**—One bowl of soup generally contains more sodium than you should consume in the entire day.
- **Fat**—Can you see the soup shining back at you? That's fat. Avoid it.
- **Calories**—I'm sure by now you have learned that added calories means added weight and more time spent digesting—both blasting at your energy.

Please, enough with the soup. Here's a strategy—if you hate the person coming over for dinner, serve restaurant soup or make up a batch using the biggest dose of sodium known to man. If you are competing with a colleague for a promotion, bring him a nice, big container of soup from a salad bar or deli prior to his final interview.

As with food, what you choose to drink is an immediate decision. Water is as close as your nearest sink, so you don't even have to purchase anything to immediately give your energy a jolt. With regard to sports drinks, soda, juice, and certain types of soup, cut them out, for good! Although you will not be drinking alcohol during your surge week, you may add a glass or two of wine in the future, as needed. Just don't get into the habit of drinking alcohol all the time, because that is an energy depleter. As I've mentioned before, I've given you everything you need in the 7-Day Energy Surge eating plan in Part II to get you into the habit of drinking only energy-enhancing drinks.

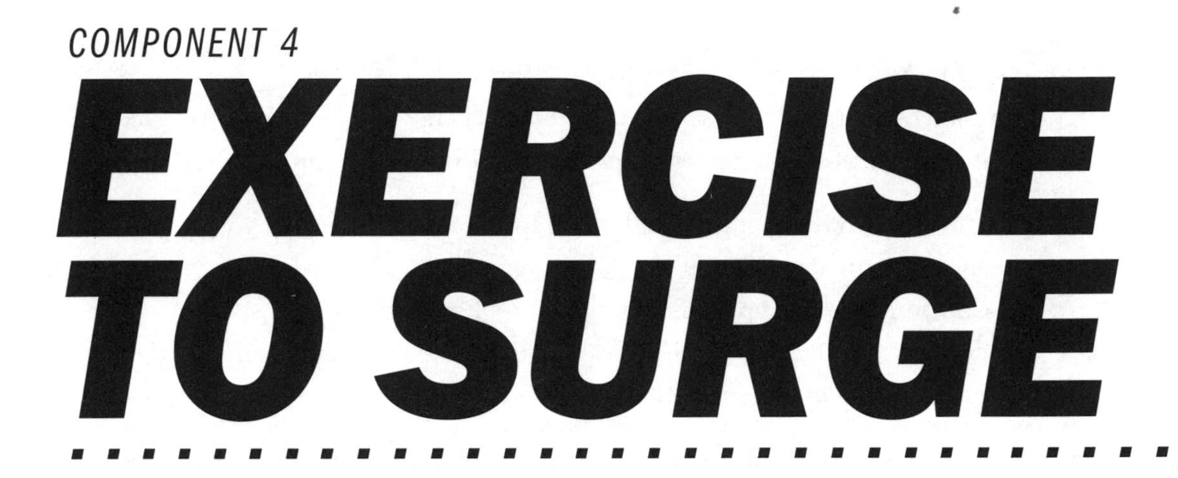
COMPONENT 4
EXERCISE TO SURGE

Most people immediately assume that exercise is hands down a plus when it comes to increasing energy. That is totally untrue, because there are some *very* popular forms of exercise that are deeply destructive to your body, your muscle, the aging process, and your precious energy. Therefore, as in the preceding chapter, I am going to tell you what style of exercise to perform more of, what to perform sparingly, and what to avoid. In general, though, remember:

More Strength = More Energy

Exercises to perform more of

- ☐ Interval strength training
- ☐ Yoga

Exercises to perform sparingly

- ☐ Classic strength training
- ☐ Pilates
- ☐ Swimming
- ☐ Walking

Exercises to avoid

- ☐ All classic, steady-state cardiovascular exercise
- ☐ Almost every group exercise class
- ☐ Crunches

EXERCISES TO PERFORM MORE OF

INTERVAL STRENGTH TRAINING

Interval strength training is one of the most effective ways to stimulate energy. I will go one step further; if you are not going to perform the interval strength-training exercises outlined on pages 71–87, then you will impair many of the other positive initiatives you are embracing to stimulate energy. It's that important.

Ideally, I want you to devote all your precious time and energy to interval strength training, because this style of exercise provides so many "energy-provoking" benefits simultaneously. Interval strength training:

1. Improves heart health. By placing a demand on the heart rate to go up, followed by a period of rest (which, by definition, is an interval), you derive far superior heart health than with classic, steady-state aerobics. This style of exercise enhances heart rate variability, defined as the beat-to-beat variations in heart rate. The Framingham Heart Study, as well as studies conducted at Harvard Medical School and Washington University School of Medicine, has linked decreased heart rate variability to cardiac arrest, congestive heart failure, and heart disease, so enhancing it is essential, and it takes very little time.[1, 2]

Plus, enhancing heart rate variability is clearly energy positive. Think about it for a moment: Is life a marathon or short bursts of activity? Clearly, it is the short bursts. Recall the last time you were in a stadium or theater and had to climb many stairs. Do you remember seeing people terribly out of breath and having to stop at each landing to gasp for air? They are unaccustomed to performing this short burst of intense activity and are using up every bit of their energy to get to where they have to go. Where will they now get the energy to enjoy watching the game or show?

Had they exercised in intervals, they would be in infinitely better shape and could take this immediate stress with less distress. Less stress on the body clearly translates into an energy pop.

2. Maintains and increases your body's lean muscle tissue. Muscle is the body's most metabolically active tissue (remember our discussion about what happens when you skip meals in Component 2?) and burns between 20 and 36 calories per pound, per day. As we age, lean muscle diminishes:

- After the age of 20, the average person loses ½ to 7/10 of a pound of lean muscle a year. That's 5 to 7 pounds each and every decade.
- As women enter menopause, their rate of muscle loss doubles to between 1 and 1 4/10 pounds each year. That's 10 to 14 pounds lost each and every subsequent decade.

The Importance of Muscle

If you don't believe me that muscle is absolutely essential to your body, then listen to what Dr. Mehmet Oz says on page 26 in the November 2008 issue of *O, The Oprah Magazine:* "I really don't like weight lifting, but I do it because I need the muscle." Forgive me, but how can you not believe Oprah's famed wizard?

- As you approach the age of 70, you lose up to 3 pounds of muscle each year. That's 30 pounds of muscle lost each decade from then on. That's an alarming amount of loss, and for many seniors it will determine whether they live a dependent or an independent lifestyle.

Only strength training will halt and then reverse this trend. If you can believe it, cardiovascular exercise for more than 20 to 30 minutes actually depletes muscle, and you will hear more about that in the "Exercises to Avoid" category. Strength is essential and fundamental when it comes to increased energy. I know I am repeating myself, but it's that important. Here is the connection:

Increased Strength = Increased Lean Muscle Tissue

Increased Lean Muscle Tissue = Increased Metabolism

Metabolism Up = Energy Up

3. Burns calories. For those looking to lose weight, you burn more calories performing an activity that is foreign to your body than performing something that your body is accustomed to. We have to walk every day in our lives and have become very energy efficient at this. Therefore, using walking as your chosen form of exercise will not burn nearly as many calories as interval strength training will. You have to switch it up with new physical challenges, thus "tricking" your body into getting stronger, leaner, healthier, and more energized.

University of Southern Maine researchers found that weight training actually burns

71 percent more calories than originally thought and one circuit of eight exercises can burn 231 calories. If you can believe it, the researchers proved that a half hour of strength training burned the same amount of calories as fast running for the same amount of time. That's a lot more calories than originally thought because most people assume strength training is static, as in you perform one set of biceps curls, then rest for 2 to 3 minutes before your next set. I totally disagree. One should keep moving during strength training to provide enhanced heart health *and* increased calorie burn, both during and after the workout.[3]

4. Burns more calories after exercise. This is called excess postexercise oxygen consumption (EPOC). When performing only 31 minutes of interval strength training, metabolism is elevated for 38 hours. No, that is not a typo. You will elevate your metabolism for 38 additional hours by performing only 31 minutes of this style of exercise. By contrast, 31 minutes of moderate intensity cardiovascular exercise elevates your metabolism for only 4 hours. That's a staggering number and the reason why the term *exercise* should by definition immediately equate to interval strength training.[4]

The reason you burn so many calories postexercise with interval strength training is that you create a great deal of "disruption" in the body. We generally think of the word

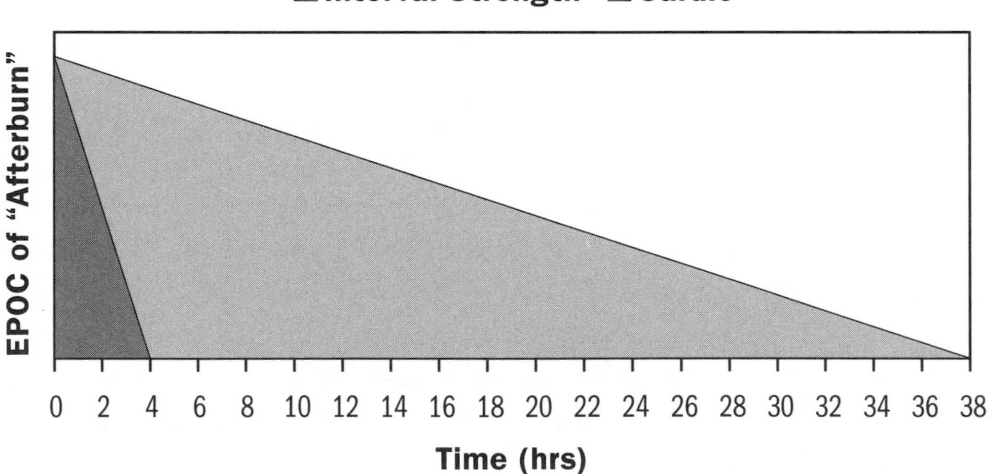

disruption in negative terms, but in this instance, it is a positive, because it boosts your metabolism by:

- Replenishing energy resources, including glycogen
- Reoxygenating the blood
- Balancing circulating hormones
- Stressing muscular tissue, which requires protein to repair
- Decreasing body temperature, breathing rate, and heart rate back to normal

When you perform interval strength training, you enhance EPOC far more than with any other style of exercise I know of.

5. Burns more fat. Canadian researchers recently reported that a mere 2 weeks of interval strength training boosted a woman's ability to burn body fat for fuel while exercising by a whopping 38 percent. That's a significant increase for those of us looking to burn some additional body fat.[5]

6. Burns more belly fat. A study from East Carolina University used probes inserted in subcutaneous fat around the midsection while the subjects performed full-body workouts (which is what you are going to do) to determine fat usage. What they found was that they burned more belly fat during exercise and for at least 40 minutes thereafter. So you not only get "afterburn," you also get "belly burn." Three other research studies published in *Diabetologia*, *Medicine and Science in Sports and Exercise*, and the *International Journal of Sports Medicine* agree.[6]

7. Enhances flexibility. When you embark upon the interval strength-training program shown on pages 72–87, you improve your flexibility. This occurs because of what is termed "reciprocal inhibition," and that means that as you contract one muscle–say, the biceps on the front of the arm–you simultaneously elongate the triceps on the back of the arm.

8. Reduces back pain. Approximately 85 percent of the American population suffers from back pain, not to mention the pain from joints that comes from injury or arthritis. By strengthening all your muscles, you take pressure off of the back and feel so much better.

The Pain-Energy Connection

I hope you realize that reduced pain is energy enhancing. Stop for a moment and think about how much better you felt when a pain you were experiencing healed itself. Or even how you feel when you pop a pain reliever. Although I am advocating fixing the problem rather than masking the pain, any way you look at it, less pain will immediately translate into more energy.

9. **Reduces neck pain.** A recent study showed that women performing strength training reduced neck pain by 79 percent, and they only exercised for 20 minutes, three times a week.[7]

10. **Seriously boosts testosterone levels.** Finnish scientists found that lifting weights increased testosterone by 49 percent. This is terrific news for both men and women, because increased testosterone levels help preserve lean muscle, decrease your mortality risk, and increase your sex drive–that's good stuff (more on testosterone in Component 10).[8]

11. **Relieves depression.** Harvard researchers compared cardio versus strength training for 10 weeks and found that those who lifted experienced a greater boost in mood.[9]

12. **Translates into less time spent on exercise and more energy left for everything else.** This is an important point. We continually hear in the media, "An hour a day of exercise" or "an hour a day of activity," etc. Who has that kind of time and energy? I know I don't. When you allocate time to essential exercise, get the maximum benefit for your precious time.

And I'm only asking you for 31 minutes of exercise, three times a week. That's 1 hour and 33 minutes of exercise per week. Period!

Now look at the direct correlation between strength training and energy:

- University of Georgia scientists found that sedentary people reported significantly more energy after they lifted weights. They believe that hoisting iron leads to a release of mood-improving chemicals, which is likely the cause of the energy boost.[10]

- Other studies have shown that strength training three times a week may increase your energy level by as much as 50 percent, and it works even on the days you don't lift. WOW![11]

Finally, you will see that all of the exercises pictured on pages 72–87 are compound exercises, meaning they utilize many muscles in the body at the same time. You will feel your upper body, core (abs and lower back), and entire lower body being challenged at the same time. By doing so, you further maximize:

- **Calorie burn.** More muscle activated translates into more energy demand on the body and, subsequently, more calorie burn while you are exercising.
- **Recruitment of fast-twitch muscle fibers.** Once again, the more fast-twitch muscle fibers you stimulate, the greater the amount of calories burned during and after the exercise.
- **Use of your time.** Simply put, you accomplish more in a minimal amount of time. I know I am beginning to sound like a broken record, but you must be very efficient when you exercise. When you work many muscles simultaneously, it's akin to being on the phone scheduling a doctor's appointment as you pay bills, organize your desk, and buy three giant-size bags of dog food off the Internet, all at the same time.
- **Strength gains.** When most people think of strength training, they think of getting into a fixed-form machine, like a chest press, and simply setting the seat height, selecting a weight, and performing X number of reps. Look, I used to do that with my clients for years, but a recent study showed that using a machine that was cable-based and allowed the user to move in multiple ranges of motion provided even more benefits. The cable-based group in the study increased strength by 115 percent, whereas the fixed-form group increased only by 57 percent.

  Even more important, the fixed-form group experienced a 111 percent increase in joint pain, whereas the cable-based group experienced a 30 percent *decrease* in pain. I just finished talking about how reducing pain is majorly energy positive, so clearly a cable-based or similar program is the only way to go.[12] You will see on pages 72–87 that the Energy Surge exercise program is performed with SPRI exercise tubing, which simulates working out with cables.

Note: Ladies, do *not* be afraid that this interval strength training will make you big. Men possess 40 to 60 times the muscle-building potential that women do because of far higher testosterone levels. In all my years in the weight loss/fitness industry, I never, ever had one woman get big. On the contrary, they got lean, lean, lean. If you don't believe me, check out the April and October 2002 issues of *O, The Oprah Magazine* and look at my work with both Diane Sawyer and Gayle King.

YOGA

Some of my past readers may be surprised to hear that I am recommending yoga. In my first three books, I didn't recommend yoga, because it is not as effective as interval strength training when it comes to weight loss. But, since the theme of this book is energy, I was compelled to include the vast benefits that yoga will provide for energetic well-being.

Yoga has been around for more than 8,000 years and is a form of movement that incorporates the mind, body, and spirit. It is actually inadequate to just use the term *yoga*, because there are approximately half a dozen different styles to choose from:

- Hatha is a basic introduction to yoga where you hold the pose in a slow-paced manner; it is good for beginners.
- Vinyasa is a bit more vigorous and is based on a series of poses where movement and breath are matched.
- Ashtanga or Power Yoga is very fast paced and physically demanding as you move from one position to the next.
- Iyengar emphasizes body alignment and using props to hold the poses for extended periods of time.
- Kundalini centers on the breath, whose purpose is that of encouraging energy to flow from your lower body upward. *Note:* A Kundalini technique will be taught in the breathing component.
- Bikram/Hot Yoga is named after its founder, Bikram Choudhury, and consists of 26 poses. It is performed in a room heated to 95° to 100°F to promote sweating and cleansing. I take Bikram in New York at least twice a month and hate it while I am doing it, but I love the way I feel the next day.

Yoga provides myriad benefits for your mind, body, and spirit, including:

- Strength
- Flexibility
- Improved breathing techniques
- Focus and attention

Try different styles and different classes to find one that works for you. You can also try the sun salutation on pages 60–61, which incorporates some basic yoga poses.

EXERCISES TO PERFORM SPARINGLY

CLASSIC STRENGTH TRAINING

Although I would much prefer that you perform your strength training in intervals to enhance heart health and EPOC, there are still benefits to be derived from a more traditional approach. If you are interested in a classic program, check out the two detailed strength-training programs outlined in *The Cardio-Free Diet*. Classic strength training, whether with SPRI tubing, free weights, machines, or your own body weight, will increase strength. By now it should be abundantly clear that:

Increased Strength = Increased Energy

Note: In all three of my past books, I urged my readers to perform more classic strength training. Since then, the abundant research is proving that this new style of interval strength training shown in this book is ideal for all the reasons cited in this chapter. You are welcome to continue to use the exercise programs from my previous books, but please, incorporate many of the principles in this chapter to get even better results.

SUN SALUTATION

1. Begin by standing with your hands in prayer position.

2. Inhale, and stretch your arms overhead, palms together.

3. Exhale, and bend forward until your hands touch your feet. Then step back, bring your arms down, and straighten your body into Plank Pose, with your arms resting on your elbows and your back straight. Hold this position for a few moments.

4. Bring your knees, chest, and forehead down to the floor. Inhale, straighten your arms, and bring your head up into Upward Dog Pose. Hold this position for a few moments.

5. Exhale, curl your toes under, and lift your hips, keeping your head down, in Downward Dog Pose.

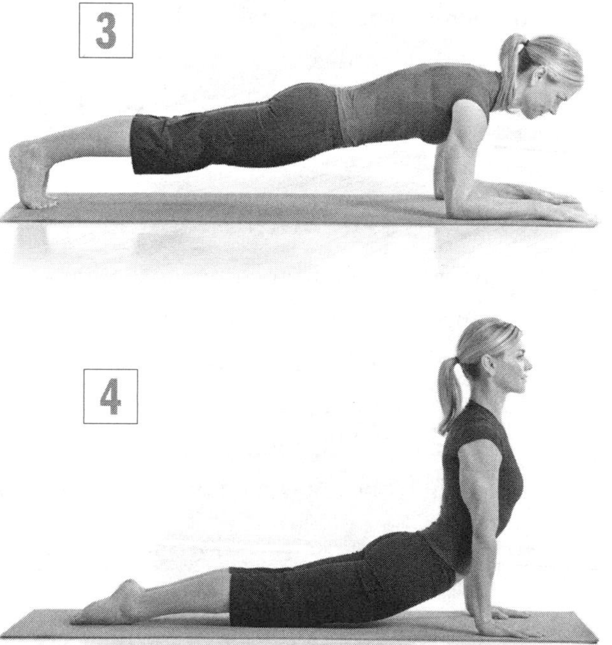

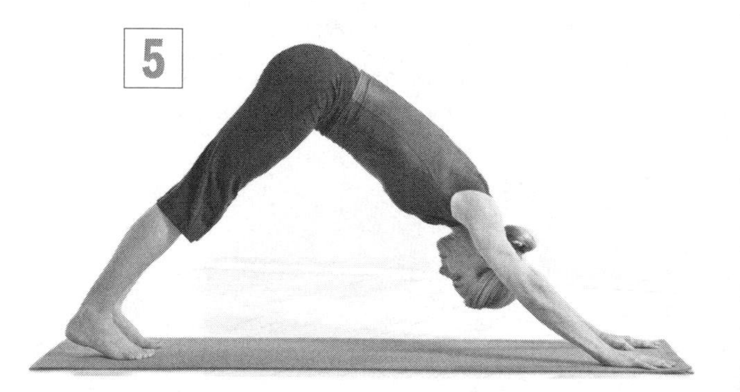

6. Inhale, bring your left foot forward in a lunge, and stretch your arms overhead, palms together. This is Warrior I Pose.

7. Exhale, twist your body to the right, and bring your arms out to the sides, but keep your head and neck facing forward. This is Warrior II Pose.

8. Bring your left foot up to meet the right, and your hands back to prayer position. Repeat these steps on the other side.

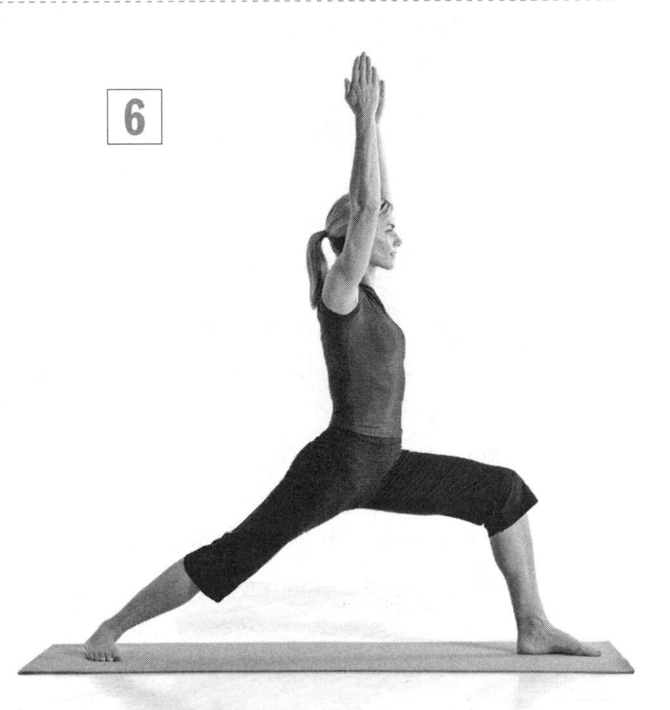

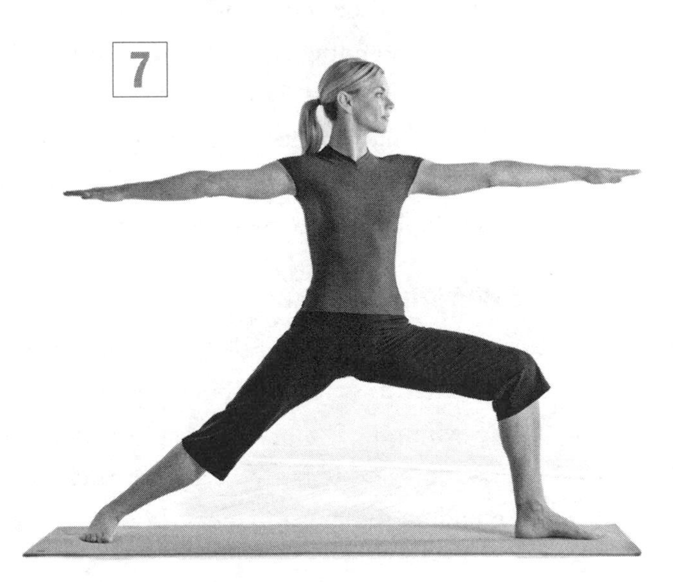

PILATES

I thought long and hard about whether to include Pilates in the "Perform More Of" or "Perform Sparingly" category. The issue with Pilates is that there are really two different forms of this discipline:

- Exercises that are performed on the floor, without any tension but your own body weight
- Exercises performed on Pilates equipment, the two most popular being the Reformer and the Cadillac

I am not a fan of the exercises performed on the floor because they remind me of Jane Fonda exercise class, circa 1970-something, and if you recall from Component 1, I instructed you to throw your old Jane Fonda tapes away. Pilates is a body conditioning program that must be taught by a qualified professional in order to reap benefits. In many gyms, though, Pilates is often taught by untrained instructors in a group exercise class, with excess repetition of movements, which can be damaging to your joints. Anything that damages your joints is going to cause pain, and we know what that does to energy.

The exercises performed on the two machines are very good for posture, core strength, and flexibility, but generally don't elevate the heart rate enough to provide heart health benefits. But many of the exercises are performed lying down. I feel that an exercise program should be more applicable to what we do in everyday life, which is why you will always be standing and working your total body on many different planes in the exercise program on pages 72–87.

If you enjoy Pilates for the reasons that I said were beneficial, fine. Would I urge you to exclusively make Pilates your energy-enhancing choice of exercise? No, because it is more of a complement to my interval strength-training program than a stand-alone solution.

SWIMMING

Let me begin by saying that I feel about swimming the way I do about Pilates, in that if you would like to swim as a complement to the interval strength training, I am cool with that. But swimming is not, in general, the best choice for elevating energy.

With regard to body weight, research has shown that swimming can actually cause you to hold on to or even increase body fat. The reason for this is twofold:

1. You jump into the cold water and your body instantly chills. A mechanism to keep you warm is to urge the body to carry more body fat.

2. You jump into the water and sink. A mechanism to keep you floating on the surface is to urge the body to carry more body fat.

Now, if you have joint-related issues that preclude you from any other style of exercise and swimming is your only option, then fine, but that pertains to a very small portion of the population.

WALKING

You will learn shortly that I am completely against classic cardiovascular exercise during your allocated "exercise" time, but I do walk everywhere. I split my time between Chicago and New York, both classic walking cities, and I try to walk as often as possible. BUT, I don't ever count that as exercise, and I call walking "active rest."

Walking just doesn't do anything to increase your lean muscle tissue, nor does it provide a great deal of heart health or cause the effective "disruption" that raises EPOC. But, I would rather you walk than get in a car, bus, cab, or train.

Exercise While Traveling

This is especially important when traveling. I log well over 100,000 miles a year in the air (thank you, United Airlines) and have simple travel rules:

- At the airport, no movable walkways, escalators, or elevators—ever! You walk and roll (your bag, that is, because you should NOT be carrying heavy luggage that throws your body out of alignment and causes injury).
- No sitting at the gate—use the time to keep moving and, at the very least, keep standing, because you are about to sit for hours on end. A recent obesity study found that obese women generally stood 2 hours less and sat 2½ hours longer each day compared to women at a normal weight. That difference adds up to 315 fewer calories burned each day. That's a big difference![13]

EXERCISES TO AVOID

ALL CLASSIC, STEADY-STATE CARDIOVASCULAR EXERCISE

Most people (with the exception of my past readers and viewers who know my position on this subject) will be shocked to hear that I do NOT want you to spend a moment of your precious time (and energy) on useless, mindless, energy-depleting, repetitive, classic, steady-state cardiovascular exercise (wasn't that a mouthful?). That's right, I don't want you to *ever* get on a treadmill, elliptical trainer, stairclimber, or stationary bike again.

As the author of the *New York Times* bestseller *The Cardio-Free Diet*, I am here to once again tell you that classic cardio is energy negative, especially when done to excess (which is how most people who perform cardio do it). Cardiovascular exercise kills your joints, posture, immune system, and desire to lose weight, because you don't burn nearly as many calories as you think. According to Duke University researchers, most treadmill displays inflate the number of calories burned by 10 to 15 percent. There is only one thing that cardio doesn't kill–your appetite. You burn a few measly calories, then eat up to twice as many because you are starving, and I hope I have clearly made the point that excessive eating is energy negative. Couple that with excessive cardio and you are chewing up your precious energy at an alarming clip. You are also speeding up the aging process.

In *The Cardio-Free Diet*, you will see that in one case study, healthy college women *gained* a pound after 18 months of cardio, five days each week, for up to 45 minutes each time. Yikes!

These are just a *few* of the reasons why you should never perform this energy-sucking form of exercise, not to mention what cardio does to your muscles. Any guesses? After 20 to 30 minutes, you actually start to *burn* muscle for fuel. Why would you ever choose a form of activity that could possibly deplete your metabolically active, strength-enhancing muscle?

Wait, I'm on a roll. Here are two more reasons to strictly avoid cardio if you desire improved health and energy:

- Increased production of free radicals. Judith Norkin, in *Life Prevention* magazine, states, "Free radicals are highly reactive molecules produced in the body, often derived from oxygen, that carry an unpaired electron on their surface, making them prone to causing damage to other molecules they encounter. The ongoing, damaging effects of free radicals may be involved in aging and degenerative disease." All types of exercise produce some degree of these free radicals. Substances called antioxidants, which are prevalent in many of the foods I recommend in the 7-Day Energy Surge, can neutralize free radicals. But with excessive cardio comes an overwhelming production of free radicals, which cannot be neutralized and will therefore accelerate aging and degenerative disease. Not so good for energy in any way![14]

- Adrenal fatigue. Dr. James Wilson, author of *Adrenal Fatigue–The 21st Century Stress Syndrome,* writes, "Normally functioning adrenal glands secrete minute, yet precise and balanced amounts of steroid hormones. But, in the presence of excessive, continuous cardiovascular exercise, the adrenals get stressed and this results in adrenal fatigue, which is associated with tiredness, fearfulness, allergies, frequent influenza,

The Research on Aerobics

A research study took a group of overweight individuals and assigned them to one of three groups:

- Diet only
- Diet and aerobics
- Diet and aerobics and strength training

After 12 weeks, the results showed that:

- The diet-only group lost 14.6 pounds.
- The diet plus aerobics group lost only 1 additional pound, for a total of 15.6.
- The diet plus aerobics plus strength training group lost 21.1 pounds and 44 percent and 35 percent more body fat than the other two groups, respectively

All that aerobics work, from 30 to 50 minutes a day, three times a week, led the second group to lose only 1 more pound. Clearly, the strength training group was the winner, and had they performed *all* strength training (especially done my way), I know the weight and fat results would have been even more impressive.[15]

arthritis, anxiety, depression, reduced memory and difficulties in concentrating, insomnia, feeling worn out and an inability to lose weight."[16]

Reread that list if you need to and realize that tiredness, frequent flu, arthritis, anxiety, depression, bad memory, poor concentration, feeling worn out, and being unable to lose weight are a nuclear *bomb* to your energy. Cut it out. Now!

Again, if you want more reasons not to perform cardio, take a look at a copy of *The Cardio-Free Diet,* as my argument in the book is even more compelling.

Note: There are many people who strenuously disagree with my position on classic cardio and are close to ideal weight. What they neglect to realize is that:

- Excessive eating ages the body.
- Excessive cardio ages the body.
- Excessive eating and cardio zap energy.

Therefore, if you are at a close-to-ideal weight by performing lots and lots of cardio and eating to accommodate that activity, congratulate yourself for successfully aging your

Why I Hate Marathons

ALL marathons should be abolished, because they are seriously damaging to the body *and* to your energy. The human body was meant to run when presented with extreme danger, as in being chased by a tiger and running for your life, but that does *not* translate into running for 26.2 miles at a steady state in a straight line on a punishing, hard surface, not to mention the excessive training required to prepare for this ludicrous event. Think about that for a moment. It makes NO sense. Plus, exercising outside in heavily trafficked or polluted areas (hello, downtown Chicago, New York, LA, San Francisco, etc.) is so horrendous that you might as well just put your mouth over a car's exhaust pipe and breathe in, because you are gulping down alarming quantities of poisonous, foul air. Finally, according to the *Scandinavian Journal of Medicine & Science in Sports*, 18 percent of those running a marathon sustain lower-body injuries.[17] Not great for your body—injury, that is—and a surefire way to destroy your precious energy. STOP all marathons. They should be outlawed!

body. See you in your sixties, seventies, and, if you are lucky, eighties. I'll be the one without the hip replacement, facelift, walker, cane, or wheelchair. I also will be the one without the leatherlike skin.

ALMOST EVERY GROUP EXERCISE CLASS

With the exception of yoga, I feel group exercise classes are TOTALLY energy depleting, from kickboxing (brutal on your joints and whole body) to spin class (who but a sadist came up with the idea of strapping your feet into toe clips and having you hunch over the handlebars, stand up, and turn up the tension? It's sick!) to supposed "toning" classes that urge you to perform 537,496 repetitions of each exercise. How about boot camp? It was devised to prepare young men, around 18 years old, for battle. Boot camp was not meant to be experienced for any other reason, so stop it. It doesn't make sense.

Group exercise classes are to be totally shunned and avoided. If you really, really hate someone, urge him or her to take a group exercise class (maybe step) and follow it up with a nice big bowl of restaurant soup and a glass of juice!

Note: I mentioned in the introduction that I used to take energy from the participants in the aerobics classes that I was teaching. That is yet another reason NOT to take these classes, because you may be the victim of an energy vampire teacher. Translation–teacher wins, group exercise participants lose.

CRUNCHES

Crunches, like simple carbs, sports drinks, soda, juice, most soups, classic cardio, and group exercise classes, need to be abolished! Most classic crunches are a complete and utter waste of time and frequently injure your neck, shoulders, and spine. The true way to flatten your abs is to challenge and stimulate them while performing interval strength training. The key is also to overload the muscles while standing and moving your body through numerous planes, similar to the movements we perform every day, which is what optimizes your visual and structural results. Doesn't that just make sense? Does lying on the floor yanking on your head make sense? I'll let you be the judge.

Finnish scientists agree with me. They measured core muscle activation while participants

Heat and Exercise

Fatigue quickly when exercising? That may be a function of heat; exercising with a fan blowing in your direction will make all the difference, because the evaporation of sweat helps cool you off more efficiently. I overheat quickly and have to be in a very cool environment to get the most accomplished in the least amount of time.

performed many different types of exercises. They found that straight-arm pulldowns (which are your Exercise 7) work your abs better than any other option.[18]

WHEN TO EXERCISE

Over the years, many people have made the excuse that they don't have the time to exercise. Researchers at Leeds Metropolitan University in England found that getting up and exercising first thing in the morning will enable you to get 9 ½ hours' worth of office work done in only 8 hours.[19] However, it is not essential that you exercise first thing in the morning. The optimal time to exercise is the time that you will actually *do* it.

The University of Georgia further supports my theory on exercise and energy: Sleep-deprived people can increase their perceived energy by 20 percent when hitting the gym *and* reduce fatigue by up to 65 percent.[20]

WHAT TO EAT BEFORE AND AFTER EXERCISE

As I discussed in Component 2, Eat to Surge, how you fuel pre- and postworkout is as important as the workout itself. In fact, not fueling before and after a workout is energy negative. So don't forget to have a light meal before your workout, and a high-protein, high-fat snack after. And don't forget the research on low-fat milk after a workout (see page 43).

THE 7-DAY EXERCISE PROGRAM

The following exercise program should be performed three days a week on nonconsecutive days. You only need to devote 31 minutes to each session, for a total of 1 hour and 33 minutes a week. The program is a full-body workout, and therefore requires

48 hours of rest before you perform the routine again. Rest also optimizes EPOC.

Many of the exercises shown on pages 72–87 are unilateral exercises, meaning that you will perform all reps on one side first, then move to the other side. You are generally doing 10 reps on each side, so you'll have 20 total reps of each exercise.

I recommend having a clock with a big second hand in clear view.

Forty-eight hours' rest is required because you create tiny little tears in your muscles when you perform the interval strength-training exercises. Don't be concerned about the notion of "tears," because you have to break down muscle fibers by overloading them in order for them to repair and grow stronger. That is also a large component of EPOC and why you boost your metabolism by creating more lean muscle tissue. It is the whole act of breaking down and then repairing muscle that requires more calories.

Throughout these 10 movements, the entire body is coordinating itself. By enhancing coordination, you will build strength from the top down and the bottom up and effectively link the body together. We are stronger as a whole than the sum of our parts. That's why these compound movements are essential. Thcy:

1. Make us stronger
2. Teach coordination
3. Promote balance
4. Enhance mobility and flexibility
5. Establish good timing, as in turning the muscles on and off
6. Emphasize rhythm; as the expression of movement becomes easier and more fluid, the body operates more efficiently

The SPRI StrengthCord

The braided exercise tubing and the door attachment shown on pages 72–87 can be purchased by going to www.jimkaras.com and clicking on "Store." That will take you to SPRI Products, the manufacturer of this equipment, and they have put together special packages and prices for my readers.

Point number 6 is important. It's true that as a movement becomes easier, the body operates more efficiently, and that's the good news. This is what happens with walking. But the bad news is that once the body becomes more efficient, it then requires a new type of challenge, or "disruption," to force it to continually keep getting more efficient and stronger. The exercise industry refers to this as "progression."

In our exercise program, progression will occur when you:

1. Step farther away from the door. The farther you step away, the more tension you create.

2. Select a heavier, higher level SPRI StrengthCord. (It comes in five resistance levels).

3. Step farther from side to side or back. For many of these exercises, you ultimately will go into a complete lunge from a simple step. PLEASE don't try that first, because I want your muscles, joints, tendons, and ligaments to have the opportunity to develop the strength to allow you to take this exercise program to the next level.

4. Perform the exercises in a deeper squat.

5. Perform stepping lunges instead of stationary lunges.

6. Perform the exercises on one leg.

7. Shorten your rest period.

Because everyone is different and will start at a different level of fitness, I've given you all the options for progression after each exercise and will leave it up to you to progress when you feel ready for it. Don't go overboard and push yourself excessively. I can't tell you how many clients and friends over the years didn't listen to me and then overdid it, which led to injury, the end of their exercise program, and a subsequent diminished level of energy.

A Word from Our Testers

"It's been tough following the plan to a T. But I do feel healthier. My body is definitely responding to the strength training and healthier food choices. With my insane schedule of working 30 hours a week and going to graduate school full time, using the exercise tubing in my own door in my own apartment is so convenient!!! Thanks!"

—Corinn D., age 27

Note: This exercise program is specifically formulated to enhance breathing. When you open up your chest with the movement, you open up your breathing. Closed shoulders crowd your lungs' ability to expand horizontally. Quick, look down at your own shoulders. I bet they are turned inward.

When you repeatedly hunch forward, then the lungs learn to expand more vertically, and that leads to tightness in the neck and shoulders. It happens because you are tensing up to get in a full breath of air. That will lead to neck pain and less oxygen-rich blood.

In addition to opening the chest, your goal should also be to open up the hips. This is important because:

1. Flow and rhythm are enhanced by alternating sides.

2. When you step back, you are teaching the body to open up at the hips.

3. You are teaching your muscles to be more intelligent than they would be if they were just operating on single planes.

The goal is to lengthen all the muscles of your body.

I wanted to specifically thank Michol Dalcourt, an industry leader in the areas of human movement and performance training and an adjunct faculty member at the University of San Francisco, and one of my Chicago trainers, Andrew Gallagher, who holds a BS in exercise science, for helping to formulate this dynamic exercise program.

WARMUP
SQUAT LIFT—1 MINUTE TOTAL

1. Begin by placing the cord at waist height in the door.

2. Stand with your feet shoulder-width apart, with your toes turned slightly out.

3. Your hands are holding the individual cord handles straight out with your palms facing down. Keep your arms straight for the entire exercise.

4. While lowering into the squat, bring your arms down in between your legs.

5. Straighten your knees to stand up, drawing in your belly button (this engages your core stabilizers).

6. Rise up to your tiptoes with the cord extended over your head. Make sure your hips do not extend forward. Your full body should be aligned.

7. Inhale on the way down and exhale on the way up.

8. This is the only exercise of which 20 repetitions will be performed, because it is the total body warmup.

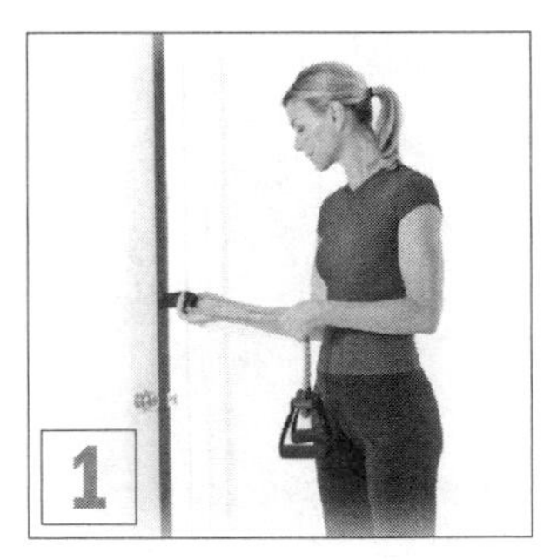

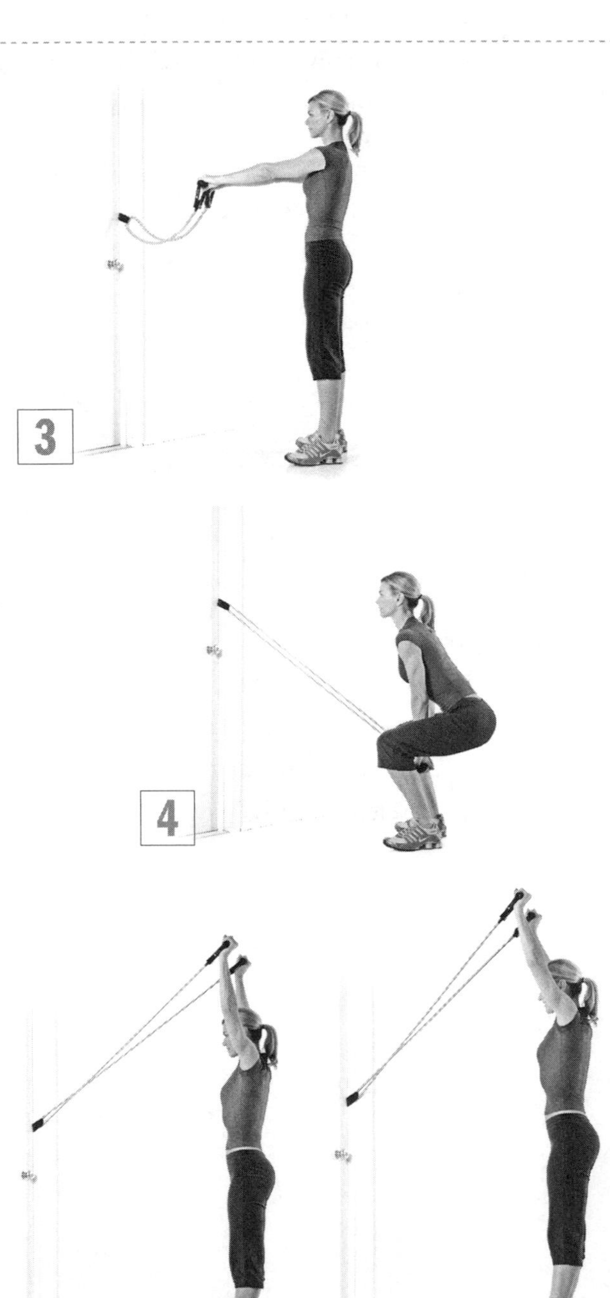

Progression

A. Stand farther away from the door to create more tension.

B. Use a heavier-tension cord.

C. As you rise up, transfer your weight to one side, bringing your hands to a 10:00 position (that is, to your left side). Then alternate on your next rep to a 2:00 position (to your right side). Always keep your head between your arms, and don't forget to come up to your tiptoes.

Note: If you find this difficult, keep your feet flat on the floor instead of rising to your tiptoes and progress to tiptoes in the future.

Rest—30 seconds

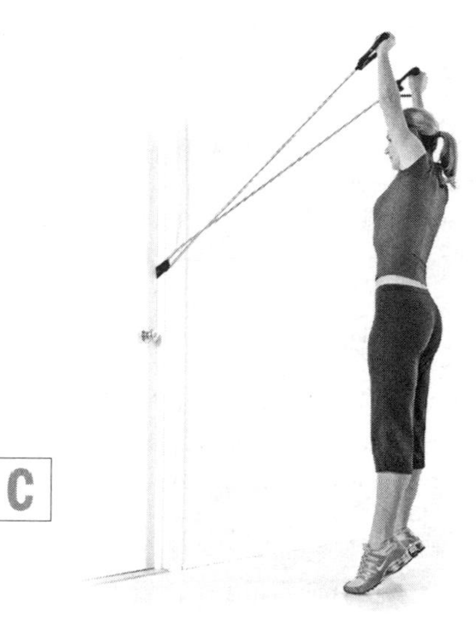

C

EXERCISE 1
SIDE LUNGE ONE-ARM ROW—2 MINUTES TOTAL

1. Keep the cord at the same place as it was for the warmup.

2. Start far enough from the door so there is some tension on the cord. Keep a wide stance (outside shoulder width) and your arms extended, but slightly bent.

3. Palms face in at all times (this is your neutral position).

4. Start by shifting your weight to the right as you slowly row the right arm back—the left stays extended while working the right.

5. Exhale as you pull back and inhale on the release.

6. Perform all 10 reps on the right arm, and then switch to the left.

7. Use a 3-second tempo as you pull, and a 3-second tempo as you come back to the starting position—each rep should therefore take 6 seconds from start to finish.

8. The 10 reps should take 1 minute to complete, then repeat on the left side.

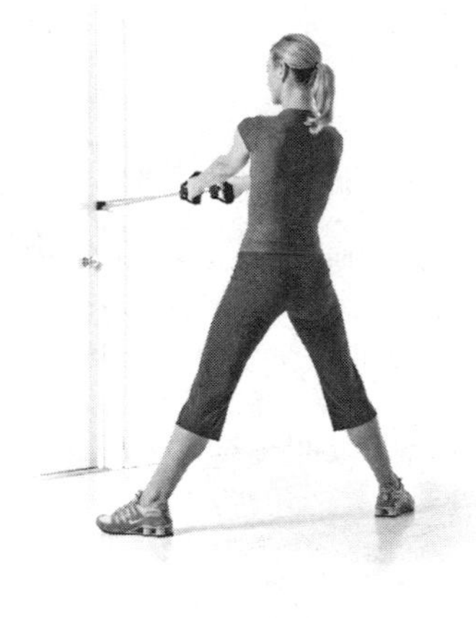

3

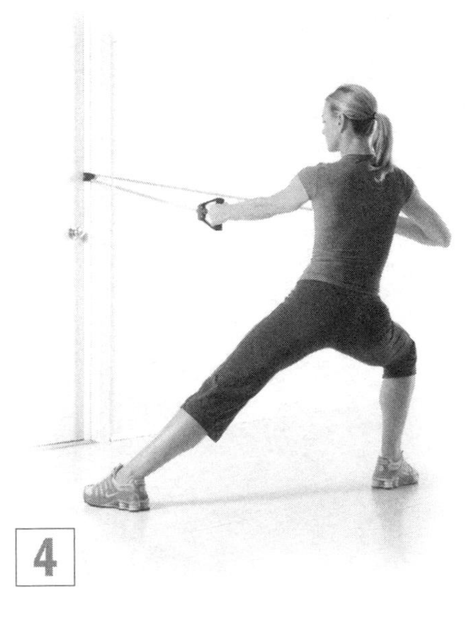

4

Progression

A. Stand farther away from the door to create more tension.

B. Use a heavier-tension cord.

C. Bring the nonworking arm into a static 90-degree position while working the opposite side.

D. Start with your feet together, and step into a side lunge with each repetition. Return to the starting position with feet together.

Rest—30 seconds

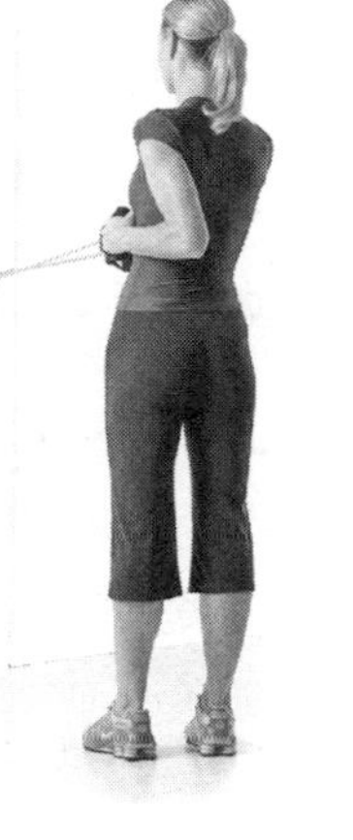

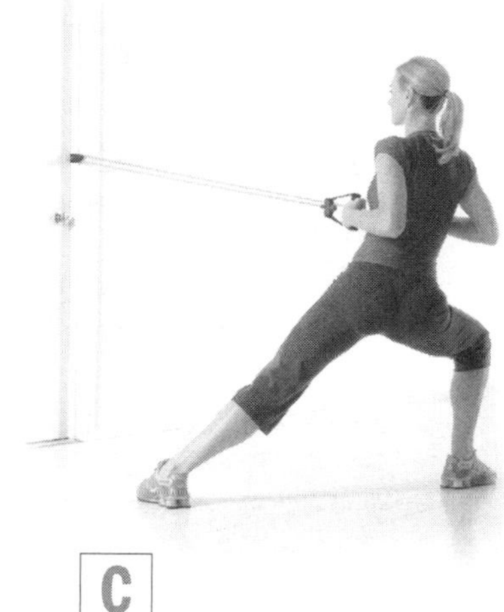

C

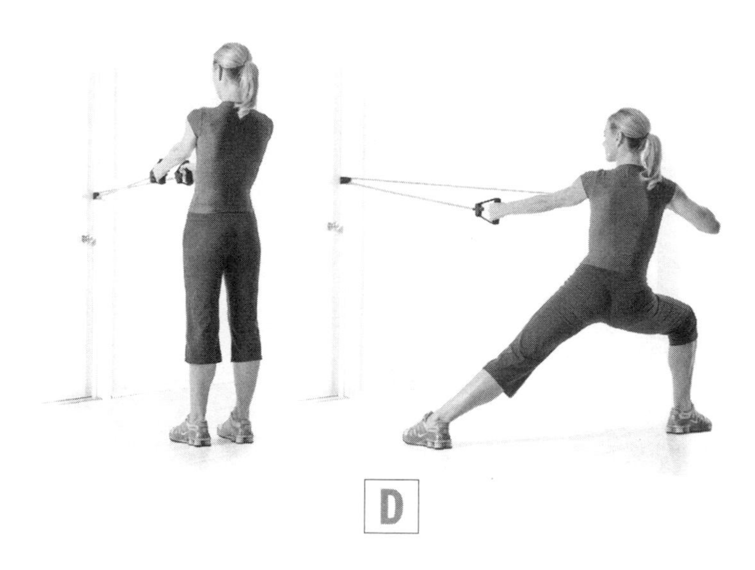

D

EXERCISE 2

LUNGE CHEST PRESS—2 MINUTES TOTAL

1. Face away from the door and take three steps to your left.

2. Assume the lunge position with the leg opposite from the arm you are working forward. The same-side leg of the arm you are working should be back.

3. Place the cord handles in each hand, shoulder height with palms down, elbows at 90 degrees.

4. Slowly lower into a lunge, drawing in your belly button. Press your right arm out, bringing your hand in line with the middle of your chest. Keep your left arm in the starting position while working the right arm.

5. Pause at the bottom of the lunge and with the press extended. Slowly return to the starting position.

6. Exhale as your arms go out and inhale as you return to the starting position.

7. Perform all 10 reps on one side, then switch both legs and arms. When working the left arm, you also want to take three steps to the right to create the same tension.

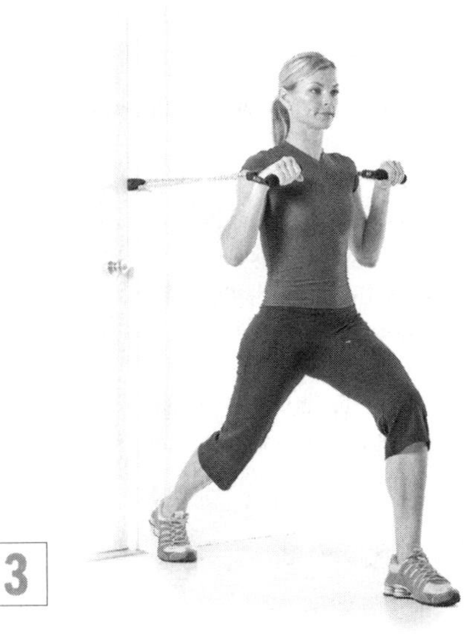

3

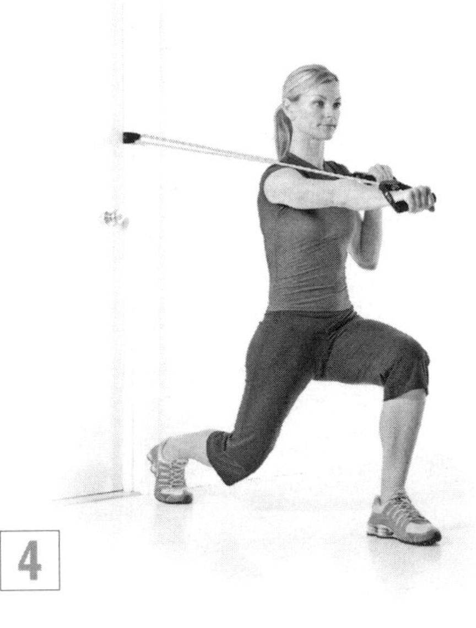

4

Progression

A. Stand farther away from the door to create more tension.

B. Use a heavier-tension cord.

C. Bring the nonworking arm into an extended static press while working the opposite side.

D. Instead of staying in a lunge, perform each rep with a forward-stepping lunge that returns back to the starting position with each rep.

Rest—30 seconds

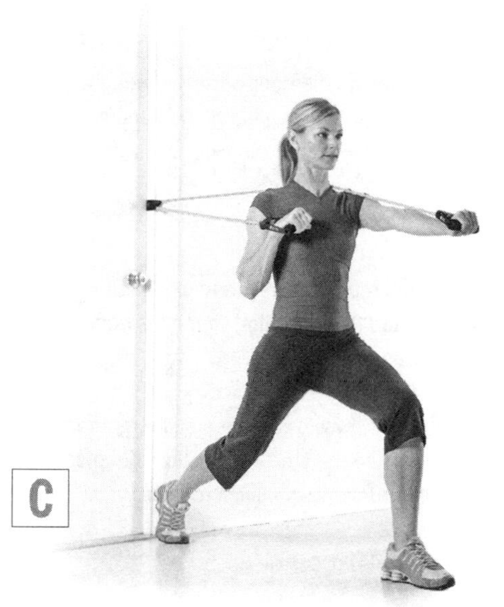

C

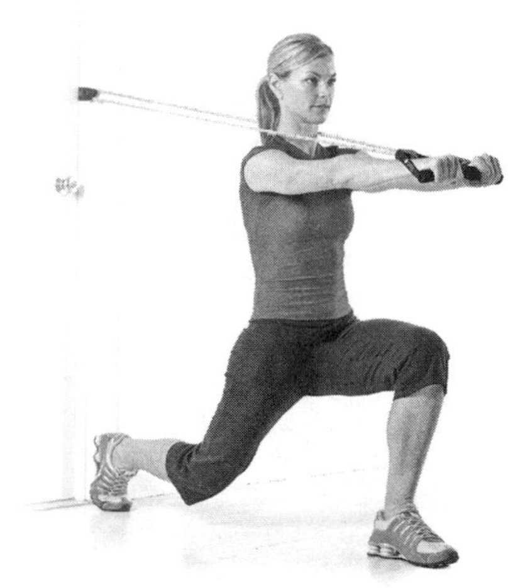

EXERCISE 3
SQUAT REAR DELTOID FLY—1 MINUTE TOTAL

1. Start facing the door with your feet shoulder-width apart. Your palms face each other and your arms are at chest height with soft elbows.

2. Lower into a squat.

3. As you return to the standing position, perform the rear deltoid fly, extending your arms completely out to your sides.

4. As you slowly lower into a squat, gradually bring your arms back to the starting position. Keep constant tension on the cord so the muscles are engaged.

5. Inhale down, exhale up.

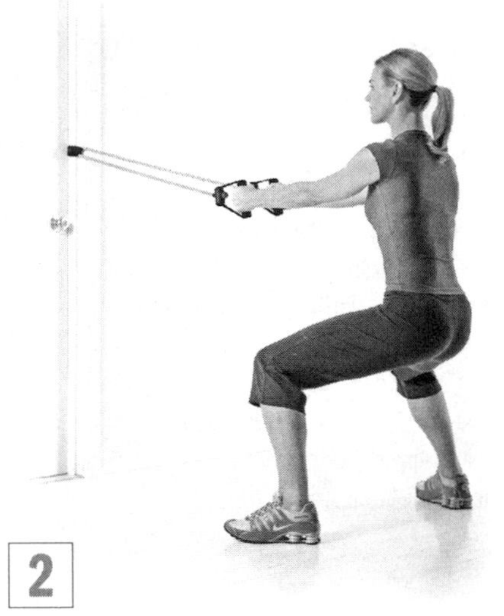

2

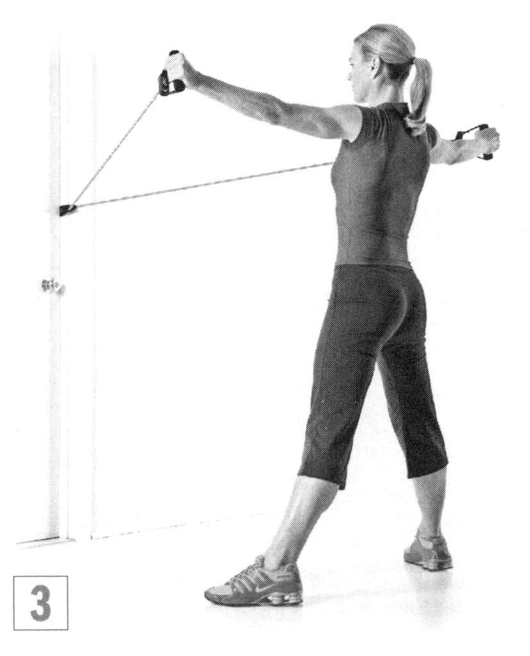

3

Progression

A. Stand farther away from the door to create more tension.

B. Use a heavier-tension cord.

C. Stay on your toes throughout the whole set.

Rest—30 seconds

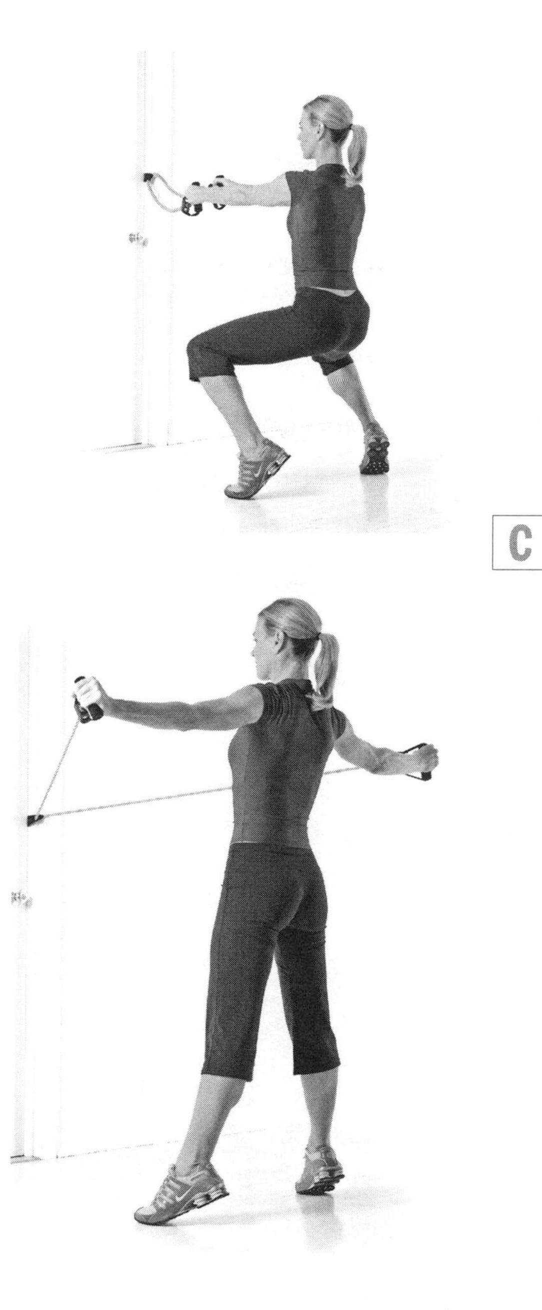

C

EXERCISE 4

ABDOMINAL TWIST WITH CHEST PUNCH—1 MINUTE TOTAL

1. Start facing perpendicular to the door with both handles of the cord in your right hand. Start with the right hand locked at the chest with your elbow up, forearm in line with the cable. Your palm is facing down.

2. Start by drawing in the belly button. Twist away from the door, pressing your right arm forward in a chest press as if you were throwing a punch. Be sure to twist from the abdominals.

3. Slowly return to the starting position.

4. This is a 2-count exercise, which is much quicker than the first three exercises in this program.

5. Perform 15 reps (30 seconds) of this exercise on each side.

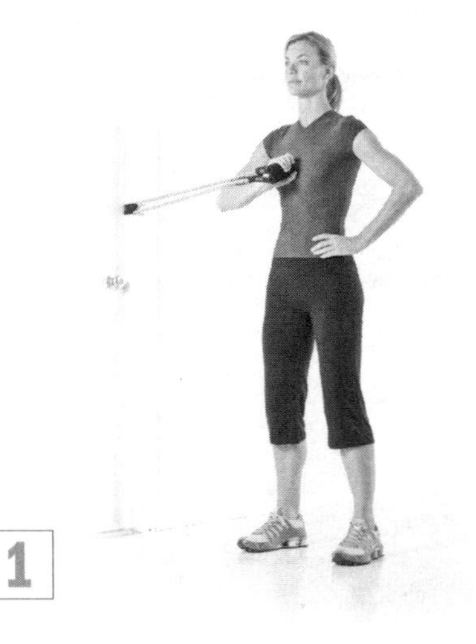
1

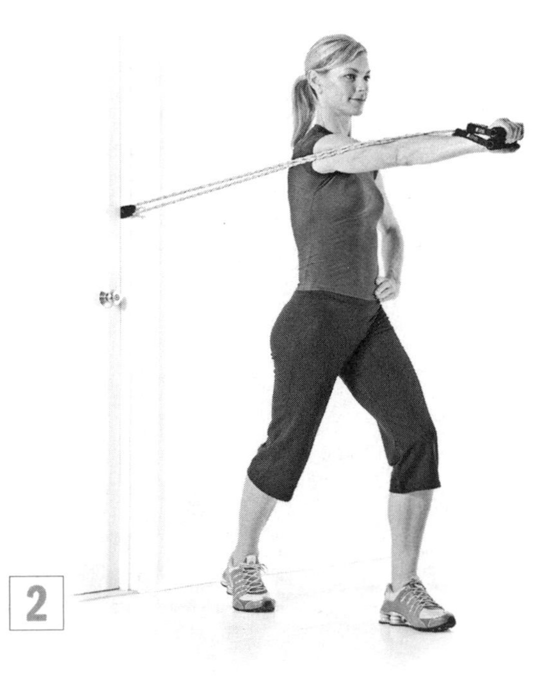
2

Progression

A. Stand farther away from the door to create more tension.

B. Use a heavier-tension cord.

C. Add more of a twist by facing the door and increasing the range of motion of the twist.

D. Incorporate a squat. From the starting position, lower into a squat.

Staying in your squat, twist away from the door and perform the chest punch. You will end in a forward lunge with your left foot forward.

Return to the lunge position.

Rest—30 seconds

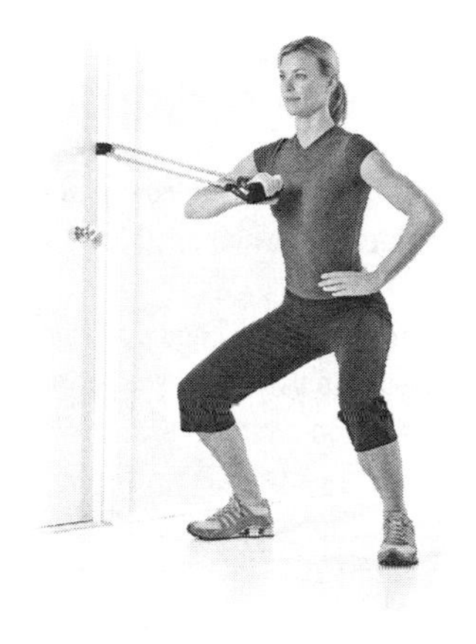

D

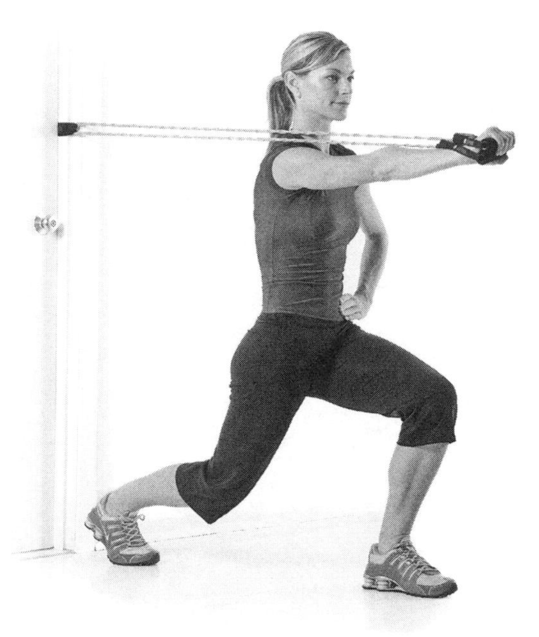

EXERCISE 5
BACK ROW WITH TWIST—1 MINUTE TOTAL

1. The cord is in the same position as in Exercise 4.

2. Step 4 feet back from the door.

3. Both handles of the cord are now in your left hand, with your palm facing down at shoulder height.

4. Twist away from the door, then pull your left arm to your chest. Be sure to twist from your abdominals and keep constant tension on the cord.

5. Slowly return to the starting position.

6. Again, this is a 2-count move, which is much quicker than the first three exercises in this program.

7. Perform 15 reps (30 seconds) of this exercise on each side.

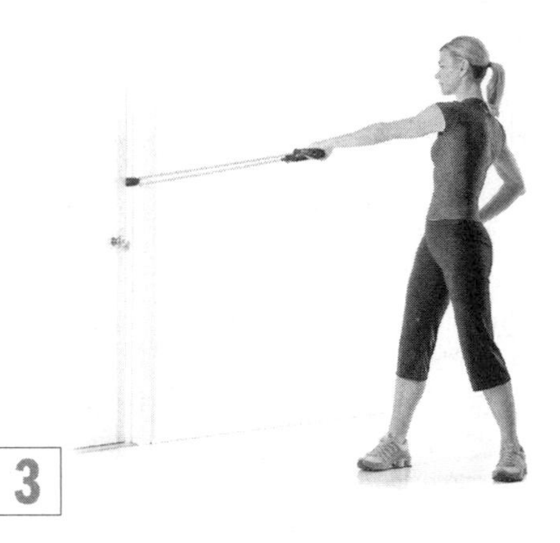

3

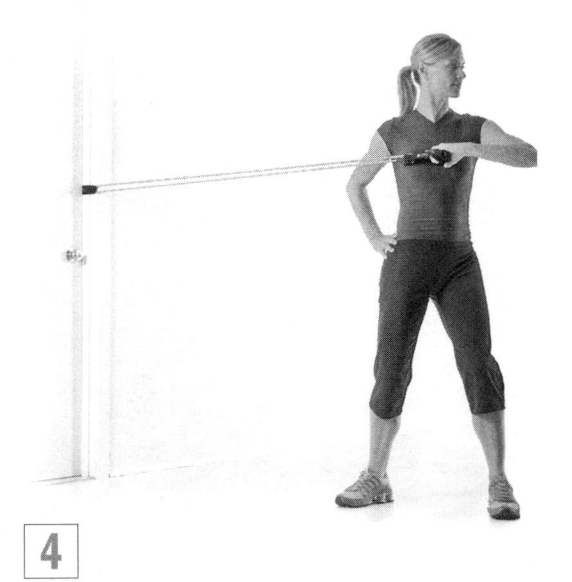

4

Progression

A. Stand farther away from the door to create more tension.

B. Use a heavier-tension cord.

C. Add more of a twist by taking 2 steps to your left.

D. Incorporate a lunge. Face the door and assume the lunge position with your right foot forward. Twist away from the door, then pull your left arm to your chest, keeping your knees bent so that you end in a squat.

Return to the lunge position.

Rest—30 seconds

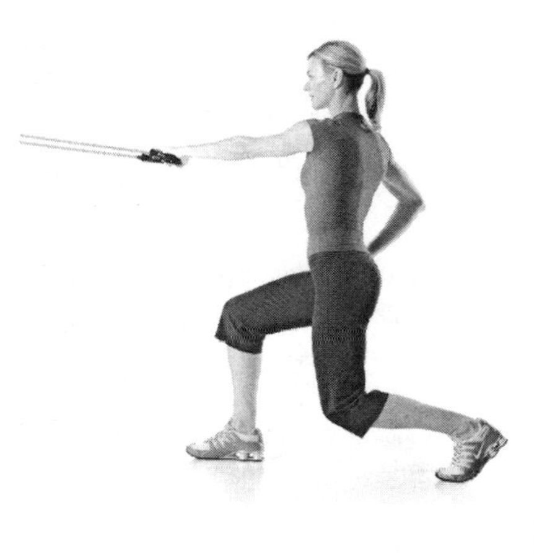

D

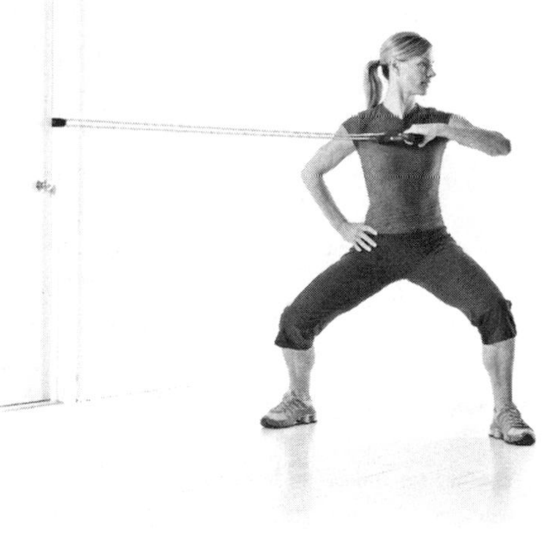

EXERCISE 6
SQUAT WITH Y, T, W, AND L—2 MINUTES TOTAL

1. The cord is in the same position as in Exercise 5.

2. Start by holding one handle in each hand, and facing perpendicular to the door with your right side closer to the door. Place your right hand on your hip to stabilize yourself.

3. Lower yourself into a squat, and bring your left arm up to waist height. Keep your arm straight and a little tension in the Xertube.

4. As you rise and come back to standing, slowly bring your left arm over your head and to the side to make one-half of the letter Y. Keep your arm straight, but do not lock your elbow. Return to a squat and bring the left arm back to waist height.

5. As you rise and come back to standing, slowly bring your left arm straight out to the side to make one-half of the letter T. Keep your arm straight, but do not lock your elbow. Return to a squat and bring the left arm back to waist height.

6. As you rise and come back to standing, slowly bring your left arm to the side to make one-half of the letter W. Keep your arm bent and your elbow about 6 inches away from your body at a 90-degree bend. Return to a squat and bring the left arm back to waist height.

7. As you rise and come back to standing, keep your elbow close to your body and slowly rotate your arm out at a 90-degree angle to make one-half of the letter L. Return to a squat and bring the left arm back to waist height.

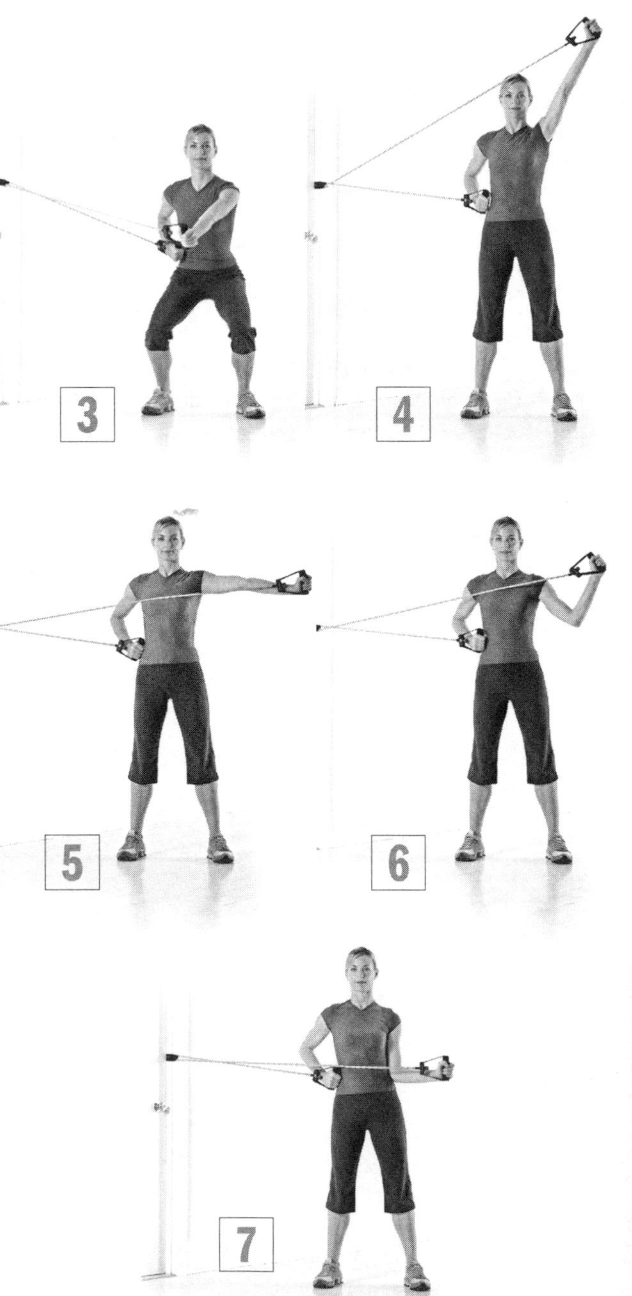

8. Each circuit is four movements (5 seconds per movement), which will take 20 seconds, so perform three circuits, for a total of 1 minute.

9. After completing the three circuits on one side, go right to the other side and replicate the movements.

Progression

A. Stand farther away from the door to create more tension.

B. Use a heavier-tension cord.

C. Eliminate the squat and perform all the reps on one leg (it's hard!).

Rest—30 seconds

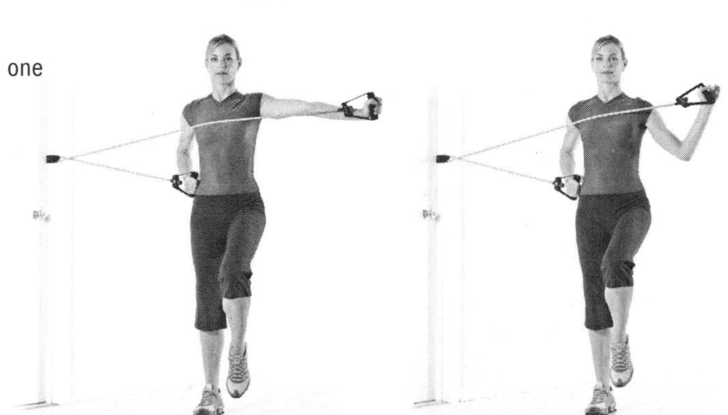

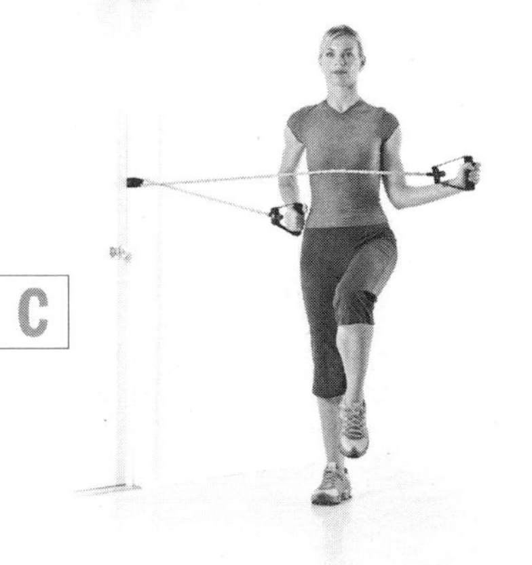

EXERCISE 7
STRAIGHT-ARM PULLDOWN WHILE SIDESTEPPING—1 MINUTE TOTAL

1. Place the cord at the top of the door.

2. Start far enough from the door so there is some tension on the cord. Your arms should be straight out with your palms facing down.

3. Step to the right into a lunge, simultaneously pressing both arms down, keeping them straight, and bringing your hands down to either side of your knee.

4. Keep your core tight; your body should be straight up at all times to fight the tension of the cord as you complete the movement.

5. Alternate going from right to left. Step back to the center in between movements.

6. Each rep should only take you 2 seconds, so perform a total of 30 reps.

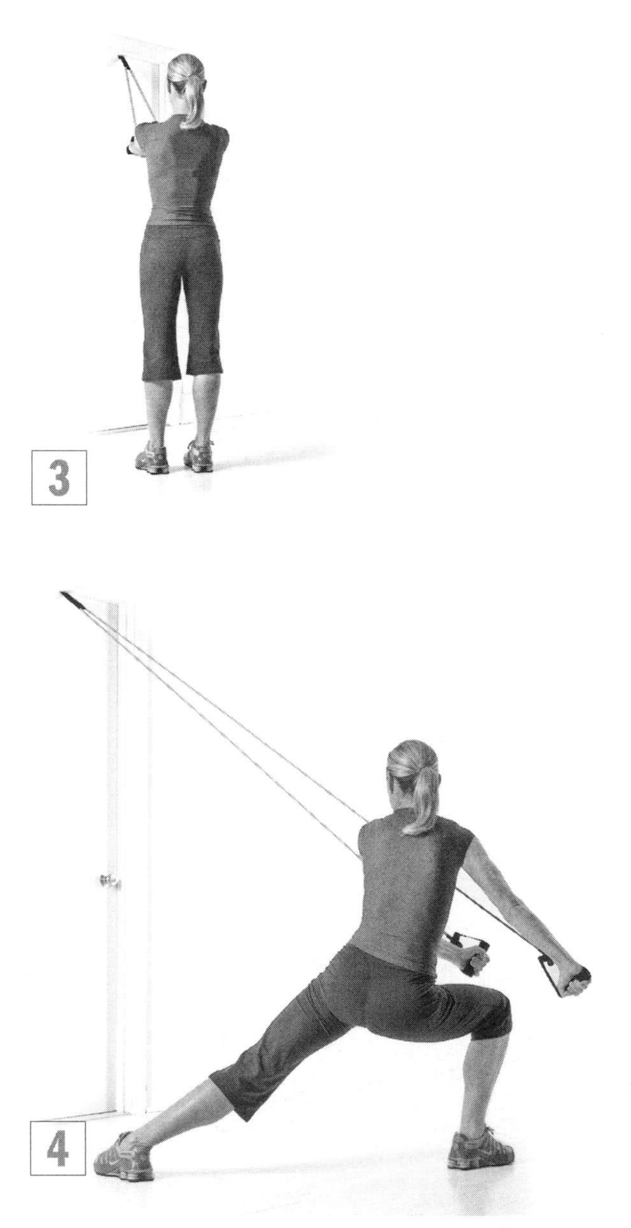

Progression

A. Stand farther away from the door to create more tension.

B. Use a heavier-tension cord.

C. Step into a longer, deeper lunge with a quicker transition between movements.

Rest—60 seconds

The total program is 15½ minutes. To reach the desired 31 minutes and maximize EPOC, you will repeat the entire circuit again, including the warmup.

As I stated at the start of this chapter, exercise is essential to a successful surge, but only specific types of exercise. If you are *still* at a place where you feel excessive cardiovascular exercise is beneficial, then please start reading this chapter over from the beginning. Your exercise mission centers around one word–*muscle.* A surge comes with strength, and strength comes with additional muscle. It's that simple.

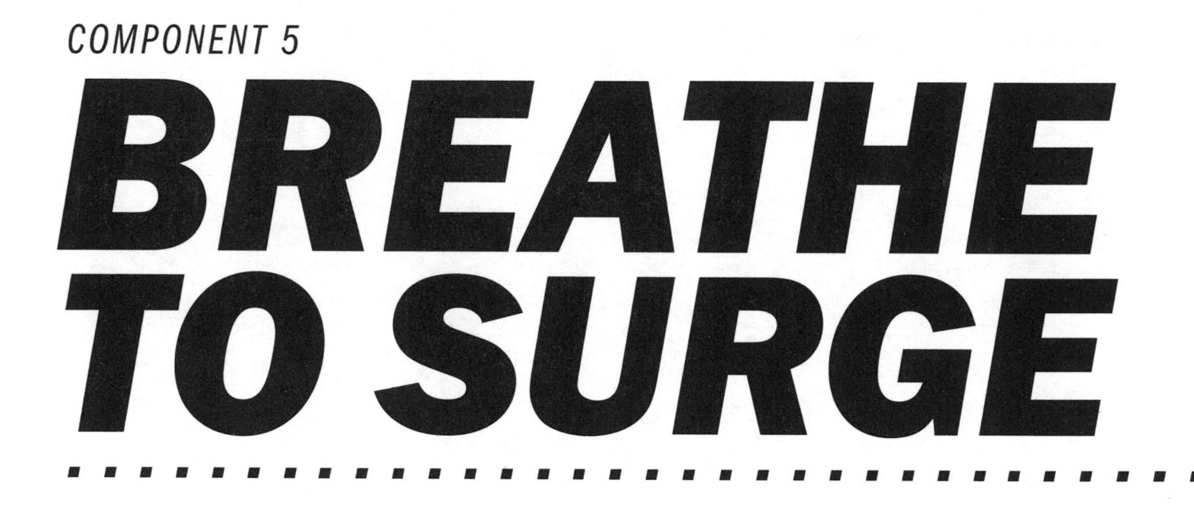
COMPONENT 5
BREATHE TO SURGE

Did you know that you inhale between 18,000 and 20,000 breaths each day?[1] If I told you I was about to teach you how to breathe, you'd probably respond that you've been doing that on your own ever since the doctor slapped you on the bottom. Breathing is both an involuntary as well as a voluntary action, and most people never think twice about their breathing from their first breath to their last.

How you breathe profoundly affects your energy. Our lungs are capable of holding 2 pints of air, but most people breathe in 1 pint or less. On average, people take between 15 to 18 breaths per minute, and a complete breath cycle consists of an inhalation of about 2 seconds followed by an exhalation of about 2 seconds, totaling 4 seconds per breath cycle. Slow, deep breathing is two to four cycles per minute versus the average of 15 to 18.

Observe others around you breathing. Notice their shoulders hunched forward from the tension that they carry in their necks and upper backs that also causes their stomachs to protrude, as the back and abdominal muscles are shortened and cannot support them in this bent-over stance. With the shoulders and neck jutting forward, there is no room for the rib cage to move upward and outward to expand because their chest is totally compressed.

For women the problem is worse, because they are taught to suck in their stomachs for that lean, long look and, to make matters worse, women's tight-fitting, metal-rimmed bras, support hose, and spandex-binding torso "tighteners" make it nearly impossible to expand their rib cage and fully breathe. Madonna did women no favors with her corset and bustier look, not to mention the infamous scene where Scarlett O'Hara is sucking it all in, to squeeze into her pre-baby frock while Mammy's yanking on her corset with brute force. It's no wonder women suffer more depression than men. I've always attributed that to hormones, never once considering that women might be starved of oxygen when dressed in tight-fitting clothes, but researchers are just beginning to link depression and lack of oxygen.

When was the last time you felt yourself breathing from the pit or bottom of your stomach? I bet it's been a long time. So here is what I want you to do:

1. Lie on your back, with your legs straight and your arms at your sides, palms facing upward (the yoga corpse pose). As you close your eyes and focus on your breath, place your hand over that part of your body that is rising with each inhalation. If that part happens to be your chest, you are shallow breathing and headed for trouble.

2. Time yourself for 1 minute and count how many times you breathe a complete cycle, defined as an inhalation followed by an exhalation. If it is fewer than 15 breaths per minute, you are in better shape than most. If it is 15 to 18 breaths per minute, dig deep into this chapter and make some changes, because this breathing rate can trigger the body's stress response. If you are taking more than 18 breaths per minute, take a huge, deep breath, do not stop, and read on.

3. Now bend your knees and place one hand over your chest and the other over your stomach, just below the belly button, and focus on allowing the breath to start in your belly and move up to your chest. If you find any tightness or tension, just place a hand over the area and gently breathe into it. Keep focusing on taking very deep breaths that cause you to feel a stretch in your abdominal, rib, and chest muscles. After 10 breaths or so, your body should loosen up and feel more natural breathing in this manner. Go back to corpse pose and feel the calming effects with your eyes closed.

THE ANATOMY OF A BREATH

The diaphragm is a horizontal sheet of muscle that separates the lungs from the abdominals and extends below your rib cage; it is crucial for the breathing process. When you inhale, it contracts, flattens out, and moves downward, creating more room for your lungs to expand. This also serves to lower the air pressure inside your lungs as opposed to the outside atmosphere. Because air always moves from high pressure to low pressure, the outside air naturally flows downward from the nostrils, throat, larynx, trachea, and bronchi to the tiny branchlike structures of the lungs called the alveoli. From there, the oxygen then travels into the tiny capillaries of the bloodstream and piggybacks on the red blood cells that carry it through the blood vessels and into your heart. The heart then sends the oxygen-rich blood to all the cells in your body and brain.

When you exhale, the diaphragm and rib cage muscles relax and move upward, now creating a decrease in the volume of the chest cavity, which creates higher internal pressure than the outside air. Now the highly pressurized air flows out of the lungs and into the atmosphere, carrying with it carbon dioxide and other wastes that need to exit your body.

Ever wonder why we yawn? Yawning is an involuntary normal process that occurs when you are fatigued, bored, or sleepy. I hope you are not yawning as you are reading this book! Because your very smart human body knows that it needs oxygen to live as well as get rid of carbon dioxide, your brain sends a message to your lungs to take a deep breath of air when it's not getting enough. Make sure not to suppress, squelch, or minimize the act of yawning. Be bold; throw your head back, open up your mouth and chest, and let it rip; let it carry your body away.

Unlike the cardiovascular, endocrine, and digestive systems of the body that you have no control over, you do have a say in how you breathe. Speaking, singing, meditating, exercising, or playing a wind or reed instrument are all times when you are controlling and forcefully expanding your breath. If you play any instrument, play more often; if you don't, pick up an inexpensive harmonica and have some fun. I am so big on music that it has its own component (more later). I am also a fan of meditation, many forms of which use breath as a focal point. I'll teach you one such technique in Component 8.

Because we always speak on the exhalation, when you need to project or lengthen words, such as when singing, you must take greater inhalations to create and maintain the sound. Who doesn't feel better after bellowing out their favorite tune? Why has chanting become so popular in the New Age movement toward peace? Don't be shy. Belt it out, baby.

Today, pulmonary physicians are alarmed by the increased carbon dioxide levels in people's blood due to poor breathing habits. To make matters worse, increasing environmental pollution is upping our air's carbon dioxide levels and asthma is on the rise. Since 1984, the rate of childhood asthma has doubled.[2] In addition, many well-known physicians, including Dr. Andrew Weil, contend that "improper breathing is a common cause of illness." Not taking full, deep breaths to oxygenate your blood and not exhaling adequately to rid your body of carbon dioxide puts you in the fight-or-flight stress syndrome, which you will read more about in Component 8, De-Stress to Surge. A shortage of oxygen also causes constriction of the arteries going to the brain, which explains why people are increasingly feeling nervous, helpless, and fearful.

Not to beat a dead horse, but constant shallow breathing slows internal systems, causing "brain fog," anxiety, moodiness, muscle atrophy, fatigue, decreased short-term memory, excessive adrenaline, increased heart rate, and high blood pressure—all smothering our energy.[3]

What's more compelling is the fact that our body discharges 70 percent of its toxins through breathing, while the balance is disposed of via sweat and bodily excretions.[4]

Most people are surprised when I tell them that their lymphatic system does not have a pump like their circulatory system has with the heart. Think of your lymphatic system as your body's sewage system; while the blood carries oxygen and nutrients into the capillaries, your lymph system is supposed to usher toxins away to your liver and kidneys, very much like a push-pull system. When you get sick and are sprawled out on the couch (not moving), your lymph nodes and glands swell as they fill up with toxins and waste. Dr. Jack Shield, a pioneer lymphologist from the Santa Barbara Clinic, placed cameras inside the body and found that deep breathing "stimulated the lymph system by creating a vacuum effect, which sucked the lymph through the bloodstream fifteen times faster than normal."[5]

THE BENEFITS OF DEEP BREATHING

Breathing with attention and awareness is key to health, happiness, peace, and energy, so learning how to breathe correctly is a must. The research on the positive effects of deep breathing is compelling; you can do it anywhere and everywhere–so fill your belly up and read on.

- Many cancer researchers claim that cancer cells cannot flourish in a well-oxygenated environment.[6] "Hypoxia is defined as a decrease in available oxygen reaching the tissues of the body. It is linked to the pathology of cancer, cardiovascular disease and stroke, the leading causes of death in the United States"[7] one study found. It has also been said that tumors grow more readily in a low-oxygen environment.[8]
- A study was conducted in Holland where one group of heart attack patients was taught deep breathing while the second group received no training. The group that performed deep-breathing techniques suffered no further heart attacks, while more than 58 percent of the second group had a subsequent heart attack over the next 2 years.[9]
- At West Virginia University, researchers noted that 10 minutes a day of focused breathing can reduce stress by up to 44 percent.[10]
- University of Rhode Island research study participants were able to reduce caloric intake by 10 percent by mindfully breathing between bites. Ten percent is a BIG number over time, and you remember how hugely energy positive weight loss is to your surge.[11]

CYNTHIA'S CORNER

One of the first things I do during an initial session with a client is assess his or her breathing pattern. With each and every inhalation and exhalation, your body is coordinating your heart rate, blood pressure, and arterial and venous dilation/constriction. If shallow breathing exists, which is usually the case except for devout yoga practitioners, I start there, because lack of oxygen causes and fuels anxiety, confusion, depression, and fatigue.

What's interesting is that when clients have adequately expressed themselves by talking it out, crying, or focusing on where they hold issues in their bodies, I always notice them taking a huge breath of air, which signals to me a discharge of tension, usually followed by a sense of calm, peace, and sometimes deep insight. When I see the client's chest and belly expanding with air, I know that the client is ready to problem-solve. I have also noticed that when I offer a suggestion or insight that feels right to my client, this full-body gulp of air also occurs, almost like a signal for the client to pause and take it all in—a physical confirmation.

For some clients, the entire session may revolve around breathing. These days, I've come to find that even children are holding their breath in the midst of fear, insecurity, and anxiety absorbed from either parents or a fast-paced, frightening world.

Breathing is our continual source of energy flow, and the good news is that we can change or reverse negative energy *and* create dynamic energy by consciously working with our breath. Surprised?

The action of full-belly breathing actually massages your internal organs and the muscles of the back, ribs, and abdomen, thus promoting a healthy exchange of oxygen. Deep breathing encourages the parasympathetic nervous system (I know that's a mouthful, but it is important because it is the one that causes you to relax) to move into mellow mode and soothe the mind and body from anxiety and/or depression. That is why exercise is an antidote for depression: It forces your body to breathe deeply.

Looking for more reasons to make breathing a priority? Deep breathing also helps you burn more body fat. When you are taxed and fatigued, your body burns sugar (glycogen) rather than fat; when you breathe and relax your body, it says "thank you" and burns fat instead.

Don't Try This at Home

One of the reasons why smokers claim that cigarettes are relaxing is because smoking encourages them to take deep breaths. Go figure! Even deep-breathing poison somehow relaxes the body.

HOW TO BREATHE

If you are not at optimum health, the good news is that you can speed up your recovery and assist your body's immune system by breathing. Eastern cultures knew about this centuries ago; yoga, qi gong, and tai chi emphasize breathing and deliver improved health, long life, and energy!

When you exhale, keep your spine straight, your shoulder blades together and down, and your neck between your shoulders; do not collapse at the heart or mid body. Be conscious of your exhalation and when you think you are at the bottom of the exhalation, gently contract your lower abdominals inward to force the stale air out.

Normal breathing alternates from one nostril to the next all day long. In a healthy person, breathing will move from one nostril to the other about every 1½ to 3 hours. When you breathe through your left nostril, your brain's right hemisphere shows increased electrical activity, and dominant breathing through the right nostril activates the left hemisphere.[13] Yogis and Eastern medicine practitioners believe that:

- Breathing from one nostril for more than 2 hours brings on imbalance.
- Too much time breathing through the right nostril promotes anxiety and nervousness.
- Too much time breathing through the left nostril brings on fatigue and lack of focus.

Western science agrees that this cycle of right to left dominant nostril breathing activates opposite hemispheric brain function. As you may know, the left side of your brain basically controls the right side of your body and vice versa. Although both sides of the brain can work together to perform many functions, the left side of the brain is associated with logical and analytical thinking as well as the ability to be more objective. The right side of the brain is associated with intuition, creativity, and the tendency to be more subjective. There is documented research that shows that when participants breathed dominantly through

CYNTHIA'S CORNER

Beverly Hills body worker and yoga master Guru Prem Khalsa taught me how to breathe and practice yoga throughout my cancer treatment. For all women wanting to be proactive against breast cancer, deep breathing can definitely help steer toxins away from your breasts. I was an expert shallow breather until Guru Prem got ahold of me. Thanks, Prem.

In his book, Divine Alignment, *Prem writes, "It is important to exhale correctly so that you can receive the inhalation. The inhalation brings in new energy but it won't take you beyond your self-imposed limits until you change your exhalation. The exhalation refines out the impurities that shouldn't be in your life and makes space for new energy to come in."[13] Prem explains that because our lower lungs have fewer capillaries than the upper portions, if you do not exhale fully, stale air accumulates, so when you inhale, the upper lungs merely recirculate that stale air. When Guru Prem teaches breathing, he starts with the exhalation.*

the left nostril, they were more creative and had better spatial skills (a known function of the right hemisphere); and when the right nostril was dominant, the left hemisphere was more active and subjects performed better on logic and verbal skills.[14, 15, 16]

Through 10 minutes of forced alternate-nostril breathing, scientists discovered that there was more of a balance between left and right hemisphere functionality as well as improved cognitive performance.[17] Yogis perform alternate-nostril exercises every day.

Anyone practicing yoga masters an awareness of their breath, and there are many different types of breathing exercises, called pranayama. Pranayama techniques help you control, lengthen, and strengthen your inhalation, exhalation, and breath retention. *Prana* means "Life Force," and the definition of *pranayama* is "control and expansion of energy," which is quite apropos to this book.[18] Remember back in the exercise chapter? Yoga was an activity to do more of. Many studies have shown that yoga breathing controls heart rhythms, lowers stress hormone levels and hypertension, calms asthma, and decreases psychological disorders.[19, 20]

A Word from Our Testers

"I really enjoy the feeling of calm, evenness, and equilibrium I'm getting from the program. I feel more aware of the breaths I take and exhale."

—Andrew M., age 41

CYNTHIA'S CORNER

Years ago, a very young Academy-Award-winning actress came in for an emergency session, suffering from exhaustion and anxiety caused by overidentifying with a dramatic role. When I asked her to lie down to breathe, relax, and prepare for a hypnosis session, I suggested she recline on her right side. Very shortly she regained composure and with tremendous clarity was able to discuss a detailed, linear plan and schedule for her mental and physical recovery. I believe it is possible that lying on that side activated her left hemisphere enough to get her out of the emotional trap that her acting had led her into.

Yoga also increases an antistress hormone (prolactin) as well as oxytocin, a hormone that induces feelings of social bonding, well-being, and coupling.[21] Low oxytocin levels have been found in those suffering from depression.[22]

The next time you are having trouble thinking in a linear fashion, having difficulty making your point, must speak publicly, or need to drive somewhere new, try lying down for 10 to 15 minutes on your left shoulder, thus allowing the right nostril to drain and open. If you want to be more creative and/or enhance your spatial skills, lie down on your right side to open up that left nostril and tap into the right hemisphere. The reasoning behind this is not thoroughly understood or empirically studied, but many informed people believe it can enhance your cognitive performance and therefore bump up that much-needed energy.

If you'd like to know which nostril you are dominant-breathing from, try placing your nostrils inside a thin glass or wine goblet and, without touching the glass, make a long exhalation. When you examine the glass you will see two moisture marks and the one that is larger is the dominant nostril, which means the opposite side of your brain is more activated. I did this throughout writing this book, as I moved my brain between the need to create and the need to edit.

Unless you are exercising or faced with an emergency, try to breathe through your nostrils as much as possible. Mouth breathing gives us too quick and too large a quantity of air, which can lead to hyperventilation and an overload of carbon dioxide, causing blood vessels to constrict and starve our cells of oxygen. The hairs in the nostrils trap allergens, pollutants, and dust to protect our lungs. The nose also warms and humidifies the air and orchestrates the proper balance of oxygen and carbon dioxide in our bloodstream.

Note: Sneezing is our body's way of expelling these particles, so blow your nose every time you sneeze and never suck mucus back in!

BREATHING EXERCISE 1

Alternate-Nostril Breathing

1. With your right hand, lightly place your thumb on the right side of your nose and your index finger on the other. Using your thumb, block off the right nostril and inhale deeply through the left nostril to the count of 4.

2. At the top of the breath, close off the left nostril with your index finger, release the thumb, and exhale through the right nostril to the count of 8. To assist in the exhalation, contract your lower abdominal muscles.

3. Now inhale to the count of 4 through your right nostril, then block off the right nostril, release the left nostril, and exhale through the left to the count of 8.

4. Do this 10 times on each side. If you find one side a bit stuffy, you can use the finger not blocking the nostril to move the skin away from your nose, creating more space in the nostril for breath.

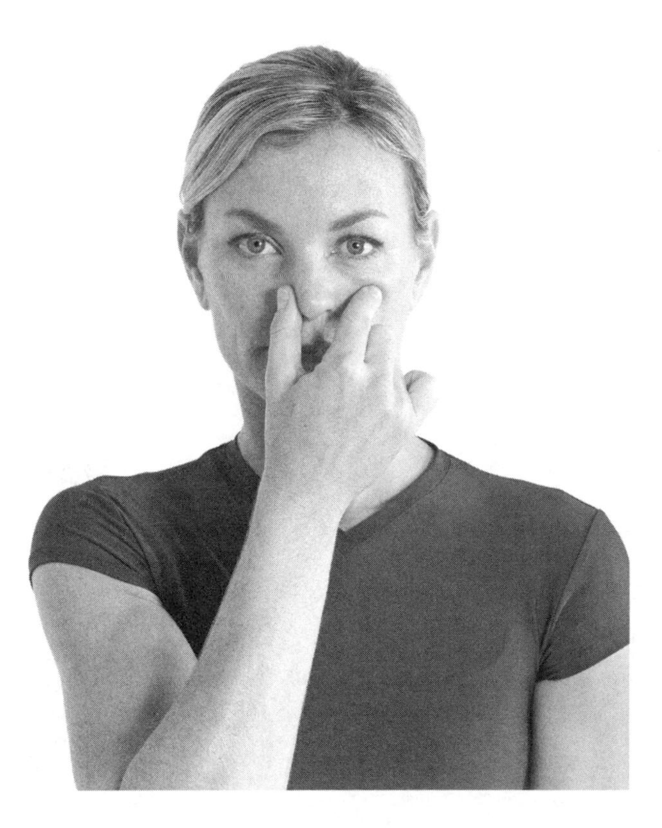

BREATHING EXERCISE 2

Breathing into Blackness

This breathing technique gives both sides of the brain a workout to bring forth creativity, logical thoughts, and a peaceful nervous system.

Note: Do not do this if you have a cold or sinus infection.

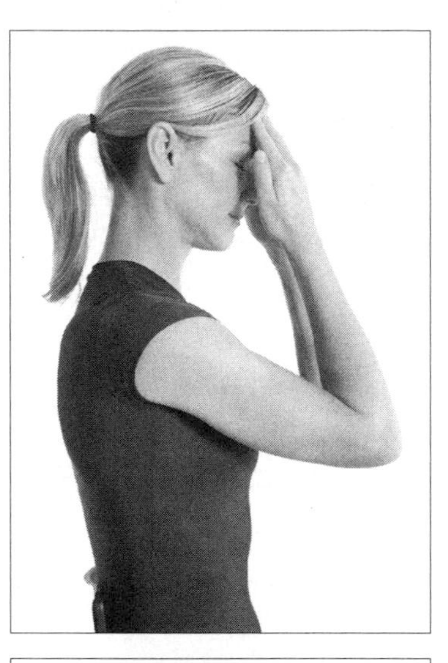

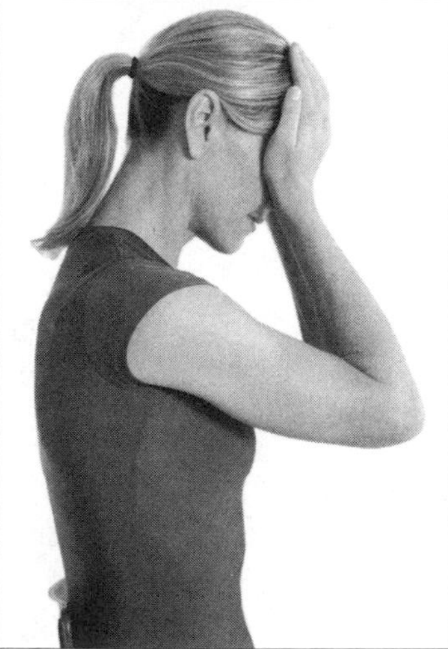

1. You can do this exercise in any position—standing, sitting, or lying down. If you are sitting, you may want to rest your elbows on your desk, kitchen table, or steering wheel (make sure you are in park). Gently place your index, middle, and ring fingers just below your hairline where there are two bumps—about 1 inch directly above the middle of each eyebrow. These bumps are called the frontal eminences and are neurovascular points that affect blood circulation.

2. Massage the bumps for a few seconds, first circling toward your nose, then away, thus bringing bloodflow to your forebrain.

3. Place your elbows on your desk or table, close your eyes, and rest each eye socket in the palm of each hand. Your fingers should be relaxed, straight, and helping to hold the front of your head. Notice the blackness and striations of light and dark. Try to make the blackest parts take over the lighter areas so that you're seeing pure rich, black velvet.

4. Inhale through your nose for a count of 4.

5. Hold your breath for a count of 4.

6. Slowly exhale through your nose for a count of 6.

7. Hold for a count of 2.

Do this for anywhere from 2 to 3 minutes and you will feel a whole new vigor. Because you want to exhale more than inhale to really get rid of the carbon dioxide, make sure you use the above ratios of inhaling for 4, holding for 4, exhaling for 6, and holding for 2.

BREATHING EXERCISE 3

Breath of Fire

This exercise is an ancient Kundalini yoga breathing practice called Bhastrika, or Breath of Fire. It not only enhances your breath but also gives you real "abs of steel." Research shows that Breath of Fire:

- Activates your brain to produce fast EKG gamma brain waves that are involved in cognitive thought, memory, attention, and problem solving.
- Provides a mild physical stimulation like healthy exercise.
- May enhance your body's ability to deal more efficiently with stress and not become so easily depleted.[23, 24]

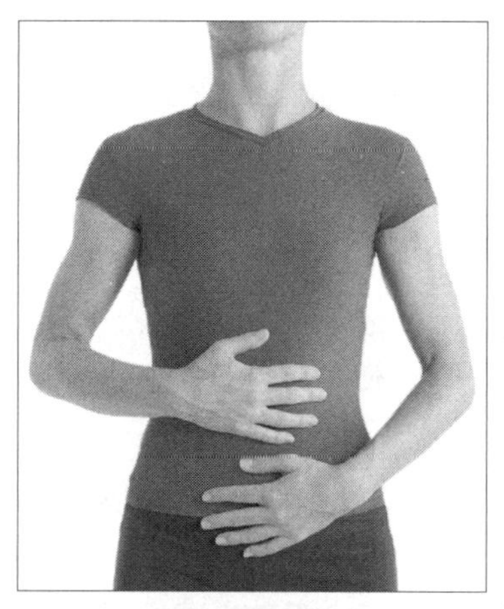

In this exercise, you are going to forcefully exhale your breath and passively inhale in a quick, rhythmic motion. Keep your mouth closed and breathe only through your nose. As you exhale, you want to contract your abdominal muscles in and upward, then down and out as you release the contraction and take an easy breath in. Start by doing this very slowly, because it is a powerful technique and can cause dizziness if done too rapidly. Start with one breath per second and gradually move the speed up to three breaths per second. Try to work up to 50 breaths at a time. The length of the inhale and exhale should be equal.

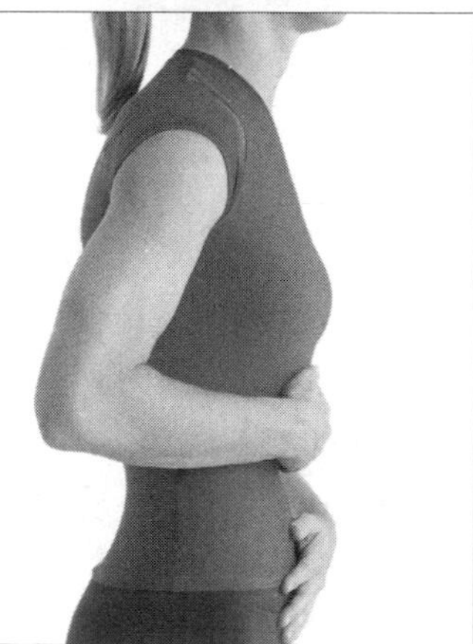

1. Start by sitting or standing with your spine erect and chin slightly tucked in. Place one hand above your belly button and the other below your belly button.

2. Exhale forcefully while at the same time making sure that your abdominal muscles are contracting in and upward.

3. Now start to inhale and feel your hands bounce outward.

4. Quickly exhale again while your hands move into your body and try to create a rhythm with the in and out breath.

CYNTHIA'S CORNER

Psychologist Fritz Perls put Gestalt therapy on the map and was a very confrontational, larger-than-life personality. He was extremely focused on the present moment in the therapy room, and called it the "here and now." He was not that interested in your past but in what you were saying, doing, and feeling right there in the room with him. Perls once said, "Fear is excitement without the breath," which makes me wonder whether by regulating and calming our minds and bodies via the breath, we could perhaps change our perceptions of life's situations from intimidating and fearful to daring and exciting.

Your hands will tell you whether you are doing this technique correctly. With each exhalation, they should be moving into your body and then outward with the inhalation. At first you will only be able to do a few breaths before you tire. It helps to keep your shoulders relaxed because there is a tendency to tighten up. After you have mastered the Breath of Fire, you can do it to music that calms and soothes you for an added element of healing.

Throughout your day, try to think of pairing your breathing with whatever activity you are doing. For example, when climbing steps–yes, climbing, not taking the elevator–inhale as you walk up the first two steps, and then exhale for the next four steps. While using this rhythmic pattern, rather than holding your breath from discomfort, know that you are inhaling and expelling air more fully and will tire less easily. For further breathing appreciation, how about taking one deep breath every time the phone rings or while stopping at a red light? Make it a habit, and before you know it you will be doing it instinctively.

At this point, I know that I have given you many assignments and exercises to follow. When I first conceptualized this book, breath was not a stand-alone component. But the more Cynthia and I dug into the research and past experience we both have had with breathing, the more essential the concept seemed to your surge. Don't walk away from this chapter thinking, "Yeah, yeah, I know how to breathe" and avoid the exercises and the research supporting them. Actually do the exercises–you'll look younger, think more clearly, and steer your body away from the stress response and toward the relaxation response, thus promoting longevity and a better quality of life.

Now take a nice, deep breath!

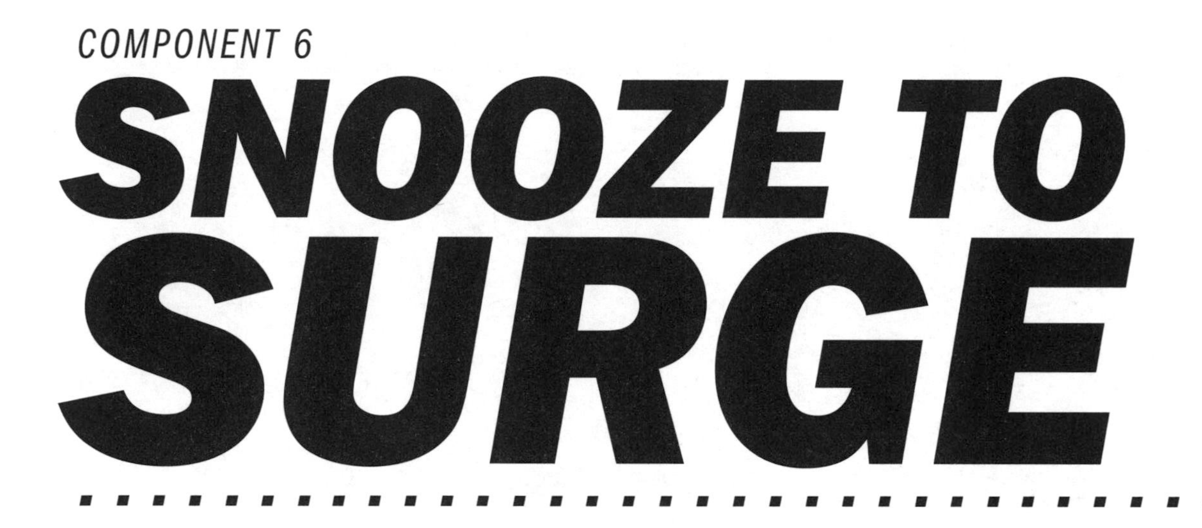
COMPONENT 6
SNOOZE TO
SURGE

These days, people brag about how little they sleep. I frequently see a CEO puff up his chest and smirk, "I get by on 5 hours a night" only to hear a peer across the room shout, "What? That's crazy! I can make it happen with only 4," and the competition begins. What, is being sleep deprived now a sign of success or a badge of honor?

Just so that we are clear, sleep is ESSENTIAL to your energy surge.

Before Thomas Edison invented the lightbulb, people slept 10 hours a night. These days, the average American is sleeping 6.7 hours a night, which is approximately 1½ hours less than 30 years ago. A poll conducted by the National Sleep Foundation in 2002 indicated that around 74 percent of the American population claim to have difficulty sleeping at some point in their life and across all ages, and 40 percent of the populace report insomnia. If you can believe it, according to Dr. Gary Zammit, director for the Sleep Disorders Institute at St. Luke's Roosevelt Hospital in New York City, "About 9 to 18 percent of adults actually suffer from chronic insomnia and aren't able to sleep for a few days or longer."[1] This is a critical issue when it comes to energy because sleep enhances so many essential functions.

Let me take this one step further. Most people are so chronically sleep deprived that they have *no* idea what it feels like to operate at normal capacity. Some just accept feeling worn out, scattered, and always tired. According to the *Sleep Disorder Special Report*, after just a few weeks of healthier sleep, some people reported feeling like "a 'whole new person,' with newfound energy (HMMMMM–there's that word again) and an improved outlook on life."[2] Many of the participants even went on to say that they now had the energy to make life-changing decisions, such as going back to school, switching jobs or careers, or even finally deciding to find a life partner. That's BIG STUFF as a result of a good night's sleep.

As I did in earlier chapters, I will now tell you:

Sleep Habits to Perform More Of

- ☐ Sleep between 7 and 8 hours a night
- ☐ Go to bed and get up within the same 30-minute time period every day
- ☐ Get up early
- ☐ Give yourself a sleep talk
- ☐ Produce, direct, and star in your nightly sleep event

Sleep Habits to Use Sparingly

- ☐ Napping
- ☐ Taking medication

Sleep Habits to Avoid

- ☐ Middle-of-the-night insomnia
- ☐ Excessive cell phone use
- ☐ Sleep apnea
- ☐ Letting your kids stay up

Before I get to the specifics, though, I want to tell you about the many benefits of getting a good night's sleep.

BENEFITS OF SLEEP

REACH OPTIMAL BODY WEIGHT

Two very important hormones related to body weight are influenced when you are sleep deprived. The first, leptin, is a good hormone that tells the body, "Stop eating. I'm getting full," and it diminishes with sleep deprivation. The second hormone, ghrelin, is a bad hormone that tells the body, "Feed me. I'm hungry." The moment you are sleep deprived, ghrelin levels increase.

Researchers from Stanford University as well as the University of Chicago found that when participants slept only 4 to 5 hours, the leptin "good hormone" went down between 15.5 and 18 percent and the ghrelin "bad hormone" went up between 14.9 and 28 percent.[3,4]

Steven Heymsfield, MD, from Columbia University in New York, states, "When you haven't had a lot of sleep, your body reacts much the same as if you haven't eaten enough," and I hope by now we know how devastating not eating is to your energy. He then goes on to say, "These hormonal changes (in leptin and ghrelin) also seem to signal the body to put the brakes on metabolism and cling to fat stores more tenaciously."[5]

Note: It is interesting that the American population has gotten bigger and bigger these past three decades as we have become more and more sleep deprived. When I give speeches to small groups and can probe into each participant's behaviors, I consistently find a correlation between weight gain and sleep deprivation. That is a total recipe for disaster with respect to your body weight, metabolism, blood sugar levels, you name it. That's strike one for energy.

Add to that the fact that most late-night grazers eat *throughout* the evening, and participants in the University of Chicago study were 24 percent hungrier. That's strike two.[6] And what do most people reach for late at night? Turkey? No. An egg? No. Nuts? No, they reach for good old-fashioned simple white carbs, such as cookies, popcorn, chips, and crackers, and that, ladies and gentlemen, is strike three. Your energy is OUT!

Need a little more motivation to get to bed? Another University of Chicago Medical Center study showed that after six nights of a mere 4 hours of sleep each night, participants were nearly brought to a prediabetic state because their insulin resistance and blood glucose levels were so significantly altered. Even after just *one* sleepless night, many of the participants had blood sugar profiles that mimicked those of people with type 2 diabetes.[7]

Plus, cortisol, a hormone that is related to stress and appetite and regulates how the body uses *energy*, spiked in these sleep-deprived participants; you will learn more about the damaging effects of cortisol in subsequent components. Hint–it decapitates energy.

BUILD MUSCLE

Midwestern State University researchers proved that, when sleep deprived, participants were able to get through their workouts, but didn't achieve the necessary testosterone boost that triggers muscle to grow. Testosterone is essential for muscle growth, increased metabolism, sex drive, and energy, and I will go into more detail in Component 10. Just so we are clear, don't do anything to sacrifice that important hormone.[8]

IMPROVE PRODUCTIVITY AND PERFORMANCE

Researchers in New Zealand and Australia report that sleeping fewer than 6 hours a night can affect judgment, reaction time, and coordination, similar to being considered legally drunk. They found that after being awake for 17 to 19 hours, individuals perform worse than those with a blood alcohol level of .05 percent. They also found that other side effects

One Bad Habit Leads to Another

According to the U.S. Centers for Disease Control and Prevention, people sleeping fewer than 6 hours a night are not only more likely to be obese, but they also have a greater likelihood of being a smoker or a drinker (or both) and are less likely to get any regular physical activity. Alcohol, cigarettes, and lack of exercise are all energy "busters."[9]

of sleep deprivation include increased depression, anxiety, stress, high blood pressure, diabetes, inflammation, heart problems, and substance abuse, all of which leach energy.[10]

ENHANCE MEMORY

Leslie Stahl (whom I have met) did a segment on *60 Minutes* on sleep deprivation and its effect on the mind and body. Participants (Leslie included) were instructed to repeat a sequence on the keyboard using their nondominant hand. After practicing the sequence in the morning, and then revisiting it in the afternoon, the group showed no improvement. After a good night's sleep (usually considered to be around 7 to 8 hours), their performance improved by at least 20 to 30 percent. This demonstrates that sleep, not time, impacts learning more effectively.[11]

Harvard University research revealed that people who were kept awake for 35 hours reduced their performance on memory tests by 20 percent. Researchers concluded that during sleep, your brain sorts through memories and stores them into other areas of the brain, making room for more input (memories) the following day. It sounds to me like sleep is the "ultimate mental organizer."[12]

LIVE HEALTHIER

University of Chicago researchers found that antibodies are weaker in people who are sleep deprived, possibly by as much as 50 percent. Get your rest, and your body is ready to fight. Skip sleep, and you leave your body in a vulnerable state. Clearly, as I have pointed out, diminished health is an energy wipeout.[13]

Plus, a 2007 University of Texas study found that melatonin, a hormone that helps regulate circadian rhythms and tells the body it's time to get ready for bed, detoxifies

So What's an Hour Less Sleep?

A Swedish study based on heart attacks found that there is an increased risk of heart attack associated with daylight saving time, when clocks are set 1 hour ahead, probably caused by sleep deprivation. The study also found that the risk decreased the Monday after clocks get turned back in the fall and people slept an extra hour. Women as well as people under the age of 65 seemed to be more affected.[14]

harmful, cancer-causing free radicals, *and* it actually creates more of these cellular "gladiators" and may even boost the power of vitamin C. That's big stuff![15]

LIVE LONGER

What about living longer? You may be shocked to learn that, as far as longevity goes, those who sleep 7 to 8 hours a night live the longest. A study conducted by the Finnish Institute of Occupational Health in Helsinki, Finland, found that:

- Men and women who slept fewer than 7 hours had a 26 and 21 percent increased risk of mortality, respectively, compared with those who slept 7 to 8 hours.
- Men and women who slept more than 8 hours a night had a 24 and 17 percent increased risk of mortality, respectively, compared with those who slept 7 to 8 hours.
- Those who frequently used hypnotics (as in more than once a week) and/or tranquilizers had a 31 and 39 percent increased risk of mortality, compared to those who did not (more on sleep aids later in this chapter).[16]

SLEEP HABITS TO PERFORM MORE OF

SLEEP BETWEEN 7 AND 8 HOURS A NIGHT

What is the magic number for optimal hours of sleep each night? It varies from person to person. Personally, I need 8 hours of sleep each 24-hour period. I can get by for a few days with 7, but to truly be at my best, 8 is the magic number, and most of the benefits I just told you about seem to be optimized when you sleep between 7 and 8 hours a night. The average American is falling short of this goal. Approximately 58 percent of us sleep between 5 and 7 hours a night.[17]

Just in terms of body weight, for instance, researchers at Columbia University in New York found that compared to those who slept 7 to 9 hours a night:

- Those who slept 6 hours had a 23 percent greater chance of obesity.
- Those who slept 5 hours had a 50 percent greater chance of obesity.
- Those who slept 4 hours or fewer had a 73 percent greater chance of obesity.[18]

On the other hand, too much sleep has been linked to diabetes, heart disease, and increased risk of death, and not more than 7 to 9 hours is recommended. One recent study showed that people who sleep more than 9 hours a night were 26 percent more likely to become obese over a 6-year period. This link between oversleeping and obesity remained constant even when caloric intake and exercise were considered.[19]

And, as we saw in the Finnish Institute of Occupational Health study, men and women who slept between 7 and 8 hours had a lower increased risk of mortality compared both to those who slept less and those who slept more.[20]

GO TO BED AND GET UP WITHIN THE SAME 30-MINUTE TIME PERIOD EVERY DAY

All sleep experts agree that the worst thing that you can do is go to bed and/or get up at all different times each day. Ideally, during the next 7 days, you should go to bed and get up within 30 minutes of the same time each day. This plan tells your body when it's time to fall asleep and when it's time to get up, and that is the winning strategy for "vavoom" energy. Just as the sun and moon have their own rhythm for rising and setting, we too must foster and respect our own rhythms to nourish energy.

Take a few minutes to schedule both sleep and wake-up times during the 7-Day Energy Surge. My guess is you have never done this in the past. We're scheduled for work, kids, appointments, etc., but never sleep. If you have to move a business or social dinner to earlier in the evening, do it. If you have to push a breakfast or meeting back in the morning, do it. Also, consider when you are going to exercise, because that may have an effect on your sleep strategy. You are going to control many aspects of this "surge" week, and proper rest is essential to the energy makeover.

Note: This includes the urge to sleep in on Saturday and Sunday. You should truly stay on schedule as much as possible. It may not sound like fun over the weekend, but you will LOVE me on Monday morning if you follow this strategy.

GET UP EARLY

A research study conducted at Queens College, Ontario, by Timothy H. Monk, PhD, found that those who get up early generally are healthier, weigh less, eat properly, exercise, and then go to bed all around the same times. That "routine" is going to optimize energy because you are clearly telling your mind and body when it needs to be sharp and when it may rest. I know that as a result of what I do for a living, I have had to learn to be a morning person, and now I am hooked on the good feeling that comes from getting up early after a good night's rest.[21]

GIVE YOURSELF A SLEEP TALK

Right before you fall asleep, tell yourself, "I am going to sleep very deeply and peacefully and I will wake up at X in the morning and feel great." Use the mind/body connection to reinforce that you are taking care of yourself and that's GOOD and SMART, and stop laughing! It works.

Just obsessing about getting to sleep will keep you from falling asleep. To alleviate that, stop using your bed for anything but sleep and sex, keep a consistent sleep/wake time (as I already urged you to do), and don't go to "The Dark Side" and focus on how you will feel the next morning if you don't get enough sleep.

Speaking of talking, in 2005, the National Institutes of Health found that cognitive behavioral therapy was just as effective as sleeping pills, due to the fact that 50 percent of those suffering from chronic insomnia are depressed or anxious. You might give therapy a chance before you reach for a pill.[22]

PRODUCE, DIRECT, AND STAR IN YOUR NIGHTLY SLEEP EVENT

Start with the set design:

- **Mattress.** How old is your mattress? Are you waking up with back pain? If it is really old, you might consider replacing it. Remember, we spend about one-third of our lives in bed, so why not make it a pleasurable experience? When was the last time you flipped your mattress? That may be the best first step to a more restful night's sleep. A few years ago, I bought a new bed and could not believe the difference in how I slept each night.

Note: According to the National Sleep Foundation, a good mattress lasts 9 or 10 years, but according to Oklahoma State University, people who switched their mattress after 5 years reported sleeping better and had less back pain. You should immediately replace your mattress if you are sinking into it or feeling pain when you get up in the morning. According to Ashish Agrawal, MD, a sleep physician at Southern California Sleep Disorders Specialists, if you are uncomfortable during the night, you may cause what's called "subclinical arousal," which leads to feeling groggy the next day as a result of fragmented sleep.[23]

Please look at the size of the mattress that best suits you and/or you and your mate. If you are bigger people in height, weight, whatever, then a bigger bed may be the best option. My new bed is a king (my first one), and I love it. I couldn't imagine going back to a smaller bed. Also, in this instance, harder does not always mean better. According to *Spine*, participants sleeping on a softer bed generally had less back pain than those who slept on a harder one.[24]

- **Pillows.** Did you take time to buy your pillows or just grab the first ones on sale? Are you falling asleep watching TV or reading, propped up by too many pillows, possibly causing a strain on your neck? Pillows are critically important to how you sleep and are frequently responsible for neck pain and headaches. A 2001 German study urges you to use a medium-firm pillow because it can significantly improve sleep over the firm-firm and the soft and squishy.[25] I also bought new pillows with the new bed and it made a huge difference in how my neck felt first thing. Also, make sure that you are not allergic to the feathers in your pillow or duvet cover.

  O, The Oprah Magazine recommends that you toss your pillows every year because your pillow absorbs hair and body oils, causing it to become a breeding ground for bacteria and dust mites. Use pillow protectors that can be washed every couple of weeks to extend the life of your pillow.[26]
- **Bedding.** Is it 100 percent cotton, so that it breathes and keeps you cool? Do you use

a top sheet in the warmer months so you can get rid of your duvet or comforter? That would be my advice.

- **Climate control.** Reduce the temperature in the room, because your body's internal temperature lowers while you sleep. That will make for a more comfortable night's sleep, and a cooler body temperature helps produce melatonin, which is the hormone that tells your body that it soon will get some much-needed rest (stay tuned for more on melatonin in a moment).
- **Clutter.** Nothing busts sleep like looking at a bunch of unpaid bills, unread memos, and clutter. Sweep it into a drawer or basket and get it out of sight. I know I have said this before, but any clutter, whether it be in your home, office, car, etc., is energy zapping.

Once the set is designed, then you need to add some atmosphere:

- **Lights.** Two hours before planning to sleep, dim the lights and use a small reading light. Candles create an ambience that tells the mind and body that it is soon going to rest and rejuvenate. If too much light comes in your windows when it is either day or night, then consider blackout shades or heavier drapery, or you might elect to wear a sleep mask.
- **Smells.** What are the best smells? Lavender, chamomile, and ylang-ylang are popular sleep inducers. I light candles all the time in my home, especially when I am ready to go to bed.
- **Sound and music.** Soft, slow-paced music played 45 minutes before sleep can help bring on the ZZZZZs according to researchers (more on music and sleep in Component 9.) But, if sound, and I mean anything from a pet or partner snoring to the street sounds outside, keeps you up or disrupts your sleep in the middle of the night, then buy earplugs, as I urged you to do in the preplanning phase.

Note: Both my daughter and I like the sound of the cars on Lake Shore Drive, which is right below us when we sleep. My son, on the other hand, says that it wakes him up, so everyone is different.

Then you need to add or subtract props:

- **Alarm clock about-face.** Turn your alarm clock so that it does not face you. According to the Hallmark Health Sleep Center, watching the clock keeps the brain stimulated and prevents rejuvenating sleep.[27] Place the clock away from you, on the floor or somewhere not in your direct sight.

- **Get Snoopy and your kids out of your bed.** According to the Mayo Clinic, 53 percent of pet owners who slept with their pets had some type of sleep disruption. In addition, many parents, especially in some cultures, have the kids in bed with them for years. I know that when my son gets in bed with me, he kicks me in the head so much that I have to get out and go to the other side and once I have repeated that three or four times, I ultimately climb into his tiny bed so that I can get some sleep.[28]

  Instead, get both the pets and the kids out of your bed. The more energy you have, the more amenable you will be to playing with them and having the patience that is sometimes required for both pets and children. That way, you all win.

Before saying "action," you need to do the following:

- **TV rating.** Monitor what you are watching right before you go to bed, because this has a direct effect on the quality and quantity of your sleep and dreams. Reruns of *Friends* or *Sex and the City* are fine, but stay clear of *Cops, The Sopranos, Bride of Chucky,* and, for the most part, the news.
- **Blue light alert.** It's not just what you are watching that's important; TV and computer screens emit blue light, which has been shown to suppress that all-important melatonin production that tells your mind and body, "It's bedtime." A Sleep and Biological Rhythms study found that volunteers who spent more time at the computer or watching TV reported that they didn't get enough sleep even if they slept the same amount as those who skipped the TV/computer ritual. Bottom line, anything that blocks melatonin production will diminish quality or quantity of sleep, and that is a surefire energy eradicator.[29] Some digital clocks also emit this light.
- **H_2O therapy.** Take a warm bath or shower prior to bed because it relaxes your muscles. Just 2 or 3 minutes gets the job done.
- **"Exercise" control.** No exercise 2 to 3 hours before bedtime unless it is some light stretching or yoga that promotes relaxation. I really like yoga, as you may recall, because it promotes just the right style of breathing to prepare you to relax and go to sleep.
- **Action—I mean sex.** Does sleep affect sex? Well, according to the National Sleep Foundation, one-fourth of the respondents said that lack of sleep was affecting their

Sleep or Exercise?

I am often asked the question, "Do I sleep the extra hour or drag myself out of bed to exercise?" The answer—exercise, at least most of the time, with the exception being new mothers or students preparing for the big exam. As I have established, exercise has HUGE energy outcomes, and you only have to do it for 31 minutes.[30]

sex lives, making them too sleepy for sex.) In addition, a study published in the *American Journal of Obstetrics and Gynecology* did find a link between decreased libido and poor sleep patterns in women between the ages of 44 and 55.[31]

How does sex affect sleep? Hmmm. I know that after "it" is over, I'm out, but isn't that true for most men? Cynthia says that sex revs most women up, but men don't know that because we are out stone cold. So from a sleep standpoint, sex helps most men fall asleep but could keep some women up. But there are many, many benefits to your energy from sex, which I will talk about in Component 10, the "juicy" chapter, so stay tuned.

During the actual sleep event:

- **Bathroom behavior.** A night-light in your bathroom is a must! If you have to go to the bathroom in the middle of the night, keep your eyes in soft focus and open them barely enough to find your way. Light of any kind, whether from the sun or artificial, activates your brain to wake up.

Note: If you frequently have to get up in the middle of the night to go to the bathroom and you do not have a physical reason, such as diabetes, for doing so, you might want to limit your liquid consumption as you get closer to bedtime.

And once the sleep event is over and it is time to get up:

- **Hit the lights first thing.** The moment you get up, reinforce the fact that it is time to wake up by opening up the shades and letting sun in, turning on the lights, or even going outside to get the paper or to let the dog out; your body will jump-start that much more efficiently. Scientists believe that the early morning light will help you sleep better that evening, because it will trigger a more effective release of melatonin later that night.

- **Strength-train.** No, this is not in the wrong category. People over the age of 60 only sleep an average of 6 hours a night. But, when Texas Tech researchers had participants (average age 78) strength-train for 6 months, they improved sleep quality by 38 percent. Oh, and these same people increased their total-body and upper-body strength by 19 and 52 percent, respectively. *Note:* There is NO reason to believe that similar improvement in sleep would not be derived by anyone at any age who regularly performs strength training.[32]

SLEEP HABITS TO USE SPARINGLY

NAPPING

I happen to be a huge fan of napping, whether it involves actually falling asleep or simply shutting off my brain for a few minutes. When possible, I love to lie down (or put my head down in my office) and fall asleep for 15 to 30 minutes. That is why I said earlier that I need 8 hours of sleep every 24 hours. It may be that I sleep 7½ hours at night, then take a 30-minute nap during the day. Most research urges you never to nap for more than 1 hour because you may fall into a deeper level of sleep and therefore awaken groggy headed.

I find a quick nap to be ENERGIZING.

Now, napping is not possible for many people, and that is why in the breathing component, Cynthia and I provided breathing techniques similar to meditation, which will allow you to rejuvenate in any setting in a minimal amount of time.

Most research shows that after being awake for approximately 8 hours, the body has a natural tendency to want to rest. Instead of reaching for caffeine or sugar, I would rather you give your body what it truly wants, a little "downtime," and that will rouse energy in the long run.

There are many people who have insomnia, and for them, napping may not be a wise option. There are other people who report that they feel worse after waking from a nap. That is why I placed napping in the "Use Sparingly" category, because you need to decide whether it is right for you.

TAKING MEDICATION

Take it easy on the pharmaceutical sleep medication. In 2004, Americans filled more than 35 million sleep medication prescriptions at a cost of $2.1 billion. These central nervous system depressants have drawbacks, including a rebound effect (which means that your body begins to fight the medication) after a week or so that further contributes to your insomnia. They are also very addictive and can cause withdrawal symptoms when discontinued, as well as dream interference.[33] Of all the most popular brands, Rozerem appears not to be habit forming. Therefore, if you are having sleep issues, it may be your best choice.

> *Note:* About 78 percent of pregnant women have difficulty sleeping, and they are advised not to take sleep medications that contain benzodiazepines, such as Valium, which are believed to cause birth defects in the first trimester.[34]

When is it okay to use sleep medication? First of all, you must consult your doctor, because he/she will know what other medications you may be on in the event there could be an interaction. Your doctor will also know which type of medication would be best for you. Do *not* borrow sleep meds from anyone. Then, only use sleep medication when absolutely necessary, because it may become addictive. Also know that certain medications are less effective if taken on a full stomach.

What about herbal sleep remedies? Here are a few that may help, but do note that there is little scientific evidence that they work and you still must consult your doctor.

- **Valerian.** Valerian is a flowering plant native to Europe, South Africa, and Asia that has been used for centuries to combat nervousness, sleeplessness, and "hysteria." The ancient Greeks used it for liver, digestion, and urinary problems, as well as nausea, epilepsy, and insomnia. The Germans used it for unruly children. It is found in pill as well as tea form. Research suggests that it can be helpful for insomnia, but the evidence, as well as the mechanism by which it works, is inconclusive. Many people report that it is helpful, and mild side effects, if any, are headache, dizziness, and upset stomach. The recommended dosage is 200 to 500 milligrams for up to 4 to 6 weeks, but, again, check with your physician.[35, 36]
- **5-Hydroxytryptophan (5-HTP).** This is used for anxiety, depression, panic attacks,

weight loss, and headaches. The body makes 5-HTP from the amino acid tryptophan, which is supplied by meat (mostly turkey) and dairy products. Supposedly, 5-HTP works by converting to serotonin (the happy neurotransmitter) in the brain, thus increasing the level. In addition, 5-HTP increases the amount of time spent in deep sleep as well as REM sleep, thus promoting more restful sleep. Although there is no recommended dosage because this is a nutrient found in the body, advised dosages range from 50 to 100 milligrams, three times a day, and it is suggested to gradually increase the dose, if needed. Side effects are reported as rare but may include nausea, drowsiness, constipation, gas, and reduced sex drive. It should not be taken with other prescribed antidepressant medications or the supplement St. John's wort. Do not take for more than 3 months. Studies are still inconclusive.[37]

- **Magnesium + calcium.** Many physicians, including Dr. Andrew Weil, believe that 250 milligrams of magnesium can help with sleep, because deficiencies in magnesium have been scientifically linked to nervousness. Some report that a combination of 500 milligrams of calcium with 250 milligrams of magnesium taken 45 minutes before sleep has a calming effect. FYI–1000 milligrams of magnesium is also a lovely laxative and, again, helps combat age-related loss of lean muscle tissue.[38, 39]
- **Melatonin.** This is the natural hormone I mentioned earlier; it is secreted by the pineal gland to help the body regulate the sleep/wake cycle. Many believe that if your levels are low, supplementation helps:
  - Decrease the time it takes to fall asleep.
  - Increase the time you remain asleep.
  - Maintain a regular sleep schedule.

  Dosages vary, but some suggest 1 to 2 milligrams an hour before bedtime.[40]

Note: Do not take melatonin if you are pregnant, under 35 years of age, or have cancer, an autoimmune disease, or kidney issues.

- **German chamomile.** Europeans swear by German chamomile, which is the most popular type of chamomile, for calming nerves, relieving anxiety, and promoting sleep. A cup of tea at bedtime or a 300- to 400-milligram capsule should get the job done for most people.[41]

Note: Do not take German chamomile if you are pregnant, have asthma, or take other sedatives or blood thinners.

SLEEP HABITS TO AVOID

MIDDLE-OF-THE-NIGHT INSOMNIA

If you are in the habit of waking up in the middle of the night, eyes wide open and ready for the day, only to realize that it's 2:15 a.m. and your alarm is set for 6:00 a.m., you know that this is *not* good for your energy. There are two probable reasons for this occurrence:

- **Alcohol consumption.** Because you are not consuming alcohol during this 7-day plan, you may find that this will not be an issue. But after the 7-day plan is over, please be very, very careful.
- **Anxiety.** People under stress lack the necessary coping skills and often wake up in the middle of the night and immediately start pondering their problems. Their minds start problem-solving in an attempt to reduce anxiety and feel in control. When you are not rested, your cognitive skills decline, and you can't possibly make good decisions.

If you wake up in the middle of the night, remind yourself that thinking will resume at X time in the morning and say to yourself "STOP." Visualize a red octagonal stop sign and tell yourself, "I will attend to you at X time in the morning, when I am refreshed and rested." If you find yourself waking in the middle of the night, try these techniques:

- Practice a few minutes of Breathing into Blackness (see page 98).
- Keep a sleep mask next to your bed and put it on or place your palms over your eyes and focus on the blackness. Tell your mind and body that you are going back to sleep. Do it!
- Don't get out of bed unless you have to go to the bathroom.
- Don't turn any light on.

EXCESSIVE CELL PHONE USE

Wayne State University scientists found that more than 3 total hours a day on the cell, which is not that much for some users, especially those who don't even possess a landline, results in less energizing, deep sleep. It's not the phone itself, but the cell signals that are causing this to happen. The author of the study, Bengt Arnetz, MD, believes that the electromagnetic waves may stimulate your brain to pump out stress hormones (there they are again), which will prevent your body from finally feeling fully relaxed. Pop in your Bluetooth, because it only emits a tiny amount of this damaging electromagnetic energy; you will then be able to properly rest and rejuvenate.[42]

SLEEP APNEA

If you are always sleepy, it is important to make sure you do not suffer from sleep apnea, a life-threatening disorder that causes you to stop breathing during sleep and decimates energy. Carrying excess body weight has also been shown to increase the odds of suffering from this condition. Fill out the following questionnaire; if you have checked more than three questions, please contact your physician and arrange a sleep study, which will require you to go to a hospital or center and have your sleep monitored throughout the night. They are generally very effective, because they identify what exactly is causing your sleep disruption.

Check the appropriate line if you experience the symptom(s) on a regular basis:

1. _____ *I have been told that I snore.*
2. _____ *I have been told that I stop breathing when I sleep, although I may have no recollection of this.*
3. _____ *I am always sleepy during the day, even if I slept throughout the night.*
4. _____ *I have high blood pressure.*
5. _____ *I have been told that I sleep restlessly, and I am always "tossing" and "turning" while asleep.*
6. _____ *I tend to sweat excessively during my sleep.*
7. _____ *I frequently wake up with headaches in the morning.*
8. _____ *I tend to fall asleep during inappropriate times.*
9. _____ *Others and/or I have noticed a recent change in my personality.*
10. _____ *I am overweight.*

_____ *TOTAL CHECKED*

LETTING YOUR KIDS STAY UP

Look, as a fellow parent *and* a single parent, I can tell you how much easier it would be to just say, "Fine, just stay up if you want to." But that would not be right for your kids or mine. Sleep is crucial to children's growth and development. Among other things, researchers at the University of Michigan's C.S. Mott Children's Hospital proved a direct correlation between lack of sleep and higher body weight. What was interesting was that all children who got fewer than 9 hours of sleep, regardless of race, socioeconomic status, gender, or overall home environment, were affected.[43] The researchers believe that it is a function of hormones, which I discussed at the beginning of this chapter, late-night eating, and lack of exercise as a result of being too tired.

Hopefully, you now realize how important sleep is to your health and energy state. Remember that there is a certain amount of preparation that will aid deep and restorative sleep. Start early in the evening to wind down. Cut out all caffeine by noon, cool it with the alcohol this week, and be careful with it in the future. Monitor what you are watching on television; keep the "soothing" music soft; put the cell phone, computer, and video games away; and read something that makes you feel happy and peaceful.

Lower the lights and thermostat. Use calming aids, such as soothing music, a warm bath, candles, light stretching, meditation, and herbal teas like chamomile, and try to go to bed and wake up around the same time each day to maintain your sleep/wake cycle.

If you are a worrier and tend to wake up in the middle of the night thinking, write down anything you need to do the next day so you give your mind the license to rest. As you turn the lights off, tell yourself that you need this time to rejuvenate in order to accomplish all your goals, tasks, and work with clarity and strength.

And remember, don't pride yourself on living sleep deprived. It's not good for your brain, health, longevity, and precious energy.

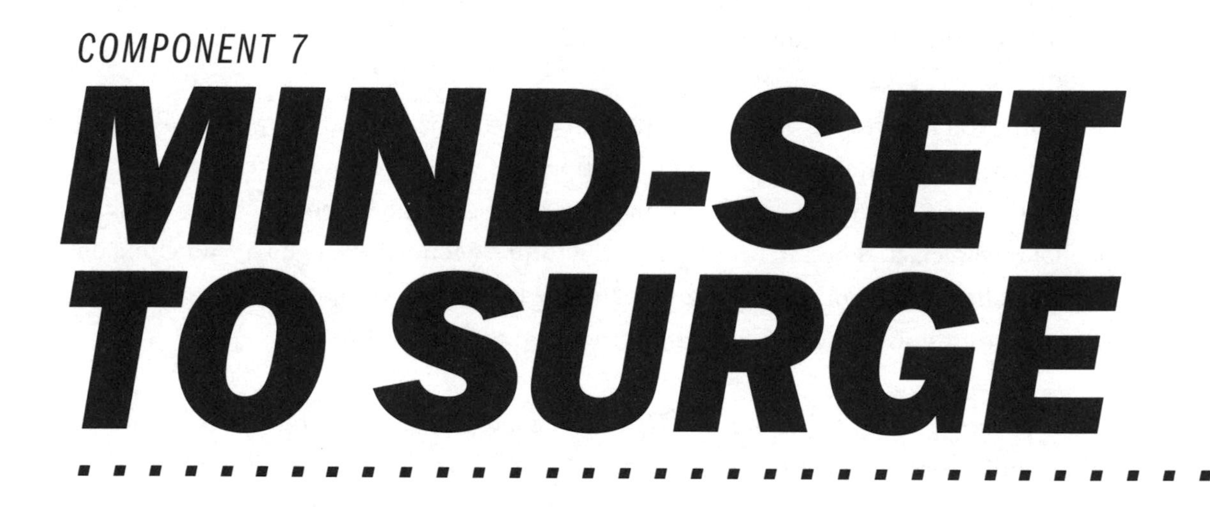
COMPONENT 7
MIND-SET
TO SURGE

Getting into the proper "energy mind-set" is critical to stoking your energy fire, creating a flow, and going with that flow. Empirical (scientific) studies clearly prove that people with a healthy, positive mind-set develop:

- More restful sleep
- Stronger immune systems
- Improved focus and concentration
- Increased confidence and creativity
- Better relationships
- Longer life
- And more ENERGY!

Someone once said, "Every step forward means leaving something behind." Many of Cynthia's and my clients dwell on their past—a true energy thief—and are therefore unhappy with their present; thinking that at their age they *should* be making a certain amount of money, *should* own their own home, *should* be successful in a career, *ought to* be married, *ought to* quit their job, *must* be pencil thin, *must* look like a model, *must* have washboard abs . . . perky breasts—ad nauseam. If they do not meet these requirements of "success" that family and society dictate, then they *must* be "losers." Sound familiar?

The renowned psychologist Albert Ellis referred to the "shoulds," "ought to's," "have to's," and "musts" as the "Mustabatory Statements." He proposed that these beliefs are driven by ego, as well as the result of really bad programming from parents, school, religion, and society. Ellis was a leader in the field of cognitive therapy and felt that antiquated dysfunctional belief systems that have us comparing ourselves with others and demanding perfection in everything we do cause us to be "absolutely miserable."

A few years before his death, Ellis was conducting a therapy session in front of an enormous audience with a therapist who had a successful practice but thought he *should* be doing better. After listening for several minutes to this therapist's misery over what he had not accomplished, Ellis bellowed, "Who gives a fu$%^k if you are not making X amount of dollars? Who told you *you* have to be making X amount of dollars to be a success? It's bullshit! You're a fallible human being. You're not perfect. Get on with it!"

The audience roared with applause as Ellis gave this man the permission to live his life—the ups and downs, all of it—without harsh judgment from himself and others. Ellis was trying to set the man free from himself. We should all strive to give ourselves a break through acceptance, empathy, and respect; few are proficient in this area, but it's a necessity for peace and happiness.

I was raised by Greek parents who drilled into me *their* measure of success—make money! Not "be a good person . . . a great parent . . . a loyal friend . . . give back to the community . . . help those in need, etc." Nope, it was simply money, money, money, and let me tell you, it's a struggle when you are given one singular variable that defines you. I considered myself a loser for *years* until I learned to reprogram *my* definition of success.

How do we block out these unwanted, relentless internal voices? How do we switch it up and do something different rather than habitually self-sabotage with the "mustabatory" statements? Ellis suggested that we start by transforming the "I must" statements into "I would prefer." That way, if you don't attain what you think you "must have" in order to be happy, then it's not catastrophic. Move on, do something different, and remember what John Lennon said: "Life is what happens to you while you're busy making other plans."

To help determine what's plaguing you, take out a pen or pencil and complete these sentences:

1. I must do ________ to feel worthy and successful.
2. I still haven't gotten over the situation when ________.
3. I am failing at ________.
4. I am succeeding at ________.
5. A good day is when ________.

Statement number 5 is important because I believe that a good day comes about by choice, not by chance. That is why each morning of the 7-Day Energy Surge you will be completing that sentence.

EVIDENCE OF THE MIND-BODY CONNECTION

After the phenomenal success of *The Secret* and *A New Earth,* it's a no-brainer these days that the mind affects the body and vice versa. When you are thinking empowering

CYNTHIA'S CORNER

These days my energy is off the charts. People are constantly asking me, "Where do you get your energy?" I'm 54, and currently juggling a psychotherapy practice, attending continuing education, speaking, and writing, coupled with being the wife of a Hollywood writer/director, caring for grandchildren, and regularly exercising. You might assume that I am run down, but to the contrary, I'm revved up. Over the years, I have come to find that abundant "life force" energy comes with a certain mind-set, a mind-set that must be cultivated and nourished. You will learn many of my tricks in this chapter.

My life journey has taught me what works and what doesn't for my energy mind-set. My journey includes being raised by strict, hard-working Greek immigrant parents, almost flunking out of college due to partying and rebellion, low-paying jobs such as cleaning houses and manicuring, opening a coffee shop, marrying, putting my first husband through medical school, reeducating myself, running my father's grocery store, catering, divorcing, moving to Los Angeles, working in the film industry, remarrying, struggling with stepkids, becoming a licensed psychotherapist, and surviving breast cancer . . . all before I turned 50!

Whether it's in my Beverly Hills practice of celebrities and the wealthy or my weekly pro bono days at a community clinic with people steps away from homelessness, all my clients complain about energy. What they all have in common is that their minds are plagued by negative thoughts, perfectionism, ruminations about the past or future, issues of control, and a tsunami of externally and internally generated stress. Stress is such a huge issue that it will be covered separately in the next chapter.

Let's face it, we've been programmed since birth with everyone else's dysfunctional views, rules, and beliefs that prevent us from making the necessary changes in our lives. Many of us live with an incessant negative mind chatter, or what Buddhists refer to as the "monkey mind." This "monkey mind" rarely sleeps; it follows us everywhere—it's automatic—it's addictive—and it's hard, if not impossible, to shut it up and toss it in a cage where it belongs. (Note: We don't want to kill the monkey because it's great for multitasking.)

thoughts–conjuring images of success, health, and happiness–you feel more hopeful and energized. Conversely, if you focus on the negatives and assume catastrophic outcomes, you probably won't be experiencing any bursts of energy anytime soon.

The big buzzword in regard to the brain these days is "neuroplasticity," and it refers to the growth and changes in the brain that involve individual cells, the connections between brain cells, or the actual changes in the physical structures of the brain. The brain and body are constantly sending each other messages through messenger molecules called neurotransmitters.

The brain uses messenger molecules to tell your heart to beat faster/slower, to tell your lungs to increase or decrease your breath rate, and to tell your stomach to begin digestion, to name a few. They also tell us when to feel anxious, sad, happy, or angry. Unfortunately, these neurotransmitters can be depleted through stress, alcohol, drugs, caffeine, and poor diet.

For the past 400 years, it was believed that after childhood the brain was fixed, except for cognitive decline in our later years. It was thought that when brain cells failed or died they were not replaced, and if the brain was damaged its structure was unchanging. But new cutting-edge research indicates that enriching, stimulating environments can actually lead to the growth of new neurons associated with new memories and learning.[1] Acclaimed author and researcher Dr. Ernest Rossi has been teaching therapists for decades about how our brains change with each activity performed. He believes that just as negativity, worry, and fear can cause our bodies to produce stress chemicals and eventually disease, so can "positive psychological experiences" bring on changes in brain structure and new brain cells that lead to "brain plasticity, problem solving and healing."[2]

I am fascinated by neuroscience and the fact that the brain is capable of manufacturing the equivalent of any drug found in a pharmacy; this can work for us or against us. Every time you entertain a thought, an idea, or a belief, your brain releases different chemicals. Each thought sends an electrical impulse across your brain that makes you aware of the thought. Psychologists found elevated levels of C-reactive protein in people who couldn't and wouldn't let go of or rethink an unobtainable goal.[3] High C-reactive protein is an indicator of inflammation and is energy negative; it's the same protein that gets lowered when we eat whole wheat and whole grain carbohydrates. So if you are obsessively pursuing a rewardless endeavor, give it up and go eat some brown rice instead.

CYNTHIA'S CORNER

Science has consistently shown how powerful the mind can be at directing and assisting in the body's healing. In my practice, after clients have verbally purged their feelings, I use guided imagery (a component of clinical hypnosis) to help them create positive thoughts and lovely chemical compounds. When I ask clients to close their eyes, move back in time, and recall happy events, within 5 minutes or so I can see their breathing deepen (you know how important that is) as their heart rate slows and their blood pressure drops. They glow and flush as their facial muscles smooth out and allow oxygen and blood to bring color to their face. Their bodies go limp, loose, and slack, and when the hour is up they truly appear much younger than when they first walked in. Just think, all these physiological responses as a result of a few moments of a positive mental state.

If you are generating angry, hostile, or sad thoughts, your brain will release chemicals that make your body and mind feel bad. Can you recall the last time you were thinking angry thoughts? Was your body loose and relaxed, or were you uptight and anxious?

Conversely, every time you sustain positive thoughts, the brain commands your body to produce the endorphins and other "happy hormones" that promote health, relaxation, and vibrant energy.

White blood cells are your body's army against infection, germs, and disease, and the actual count can be measured in a blood sample. In an experiment where healthy people imagined their white blood cells as strong, powerful sharks, clinicians found that many individuals were able to increase the number of white blood cells and their immune system's responsiveness.[4]

Renowned psychologist Martin Seligman at the National Cancer Institute is one of the originators of the concept of "learned helplessness" and more recently known for his focus and writings on positive psychology. Seligman found that cancer patients with optimism, a sense of humor, and enthusiasm had a significantly greater survival rate than those who were less positive. Humor is essential for mitigating stress, as shown by Dr. Norman Cousins and others. Studies show that laughing increases heart rate; stimulates the circulatory, cardiovascular, immune, and endocrine systems; and reduces pain and hormonal stress levels. Even medical schools are adding training in humor to their curricula.

The Amazing Power of the Mind

The most compelling demonstration I have seen of the mind affecting the body is a film of a person undergoing surgery with no anesthesia, just hypnosis. These surgeries have been filmed and documented all over the world since the mid-20th century, and it is astounding that a person can be fully awake and chatting with doctors as their surgery takes place. Irish surgeon Dr. Jack Gibson performed more than 4,000 surgeries using only hypnosis as anesthesia; some of these surgeries included amputations.

HOW TO USE THE MIND-BODY CONNECTION

THINK PREMIUM THOUGHTS

Neither Cynthia nor I believe in the concept of mistakes and often teach our clients that "mistakes" are only experiences from which we learn *and* opportunities to help us grow. Sure, we all wish we could have done things differently in the past, but when we think (not ruminate) about our pasts, we have come to realize that the greatest lessons learned in life came from losing our way, tripping, or falling flat on our faces–yes, perceived FAILURE.

General George S. Patton said, "Don't measure a man's success by how high he climbs but by how high he bounces (back) when he hits bottom." If you find yourself ruminating on a past "mistake," struggling toward an impossible goal that is wrecking your life–rather than berate yourself or pretend you are in control by obsessively thinking about the issue, try fine-tuning your expectations, desires, and feelings, and then review what you have learned as a result of this situation. As long as you are learning, there is forward movement in your life. Forward movement propels energy.

Along with forward movement comes the ability to do something novel by filling yourself up with "premium thoughts." Premium thoughts are like premium gas–high-quality fuel. Here are a few examples:

"It's not the outcome I hoped for, but I learned a lot."

"I felt like such a fool, but it won't happen again."

CYNTHIA'S CORNER

After my surgery for invasive breast cancer that had spread to the lymph nodes, I decided that chemotherapy was not an option for me, nor was ripping out all my lymph nodes. Instead, I PREFERRED to fight my disease by building my immune system with my mind rather than wiping it out with chemicals. This decision got me fired by three well-known oncologists, but I stuck with my gut feeling as well as my own research on my type of cancer.

At the same time, I knew that I had to do a lot more than just eat right, sleep right, and exercise. Each day, every few hours or so, I would take 5 minutes to visualize my white blood cells as little Pac-Men, devouring all the dark and ugly cancer cells. Your image must be meaningful to you. Recently, a cancer patient I treated visualized her cancer cells as mini devils, with pointy ears and a little tail, being speared by her army of soldiers on horseback. Each time she focused on this image, she felt more and more empowered and less helpless.

I also stopped doing things that triggered a negative mind-set, which included getting rid of certain people in my life and not doing things I dreaded. To this day, when I am tired, I cease and desist no matter what. Why, I have been known to leave a dinner party at MY HOUSE, walk upstairs, and get into bed when it got late and guests would not leave. How's that for taking care of yourself?

I have now been cancer free for 6 years and feel better than ever. The path I took to my recovery is not for everyone, and I am not recommending that you make the choices I made. Find a doctor you like and trust, and a good therapist is a must. Do your own research and discuss what additional therapies might be helpful for you in promoting healing, increasing immunity, and sustaining energy, and, of course, do everything suggested in this book!

Just as trauma and bad experiences get trapped in the brain, they also get lodged in the body. Before I work with the mind, I find it helpful to free the body up with some simple movements to help release congested energy. Getting your body to move has been shown to increase levels of dopamine (the euphoria chemical that is also increased by coffee, chocolate, and love) and elevate levels of endorphins, which calm and relax you. Mindful movements will activate your respiratory system, get a stagnant circulatory system moving, pump up the flow of lymph, activate your core muscles, increase your creative right brain's awareness, and promote a swell and release of energy.[5, 6]

"The hotel was a dump, but we laughed the whole time we were there."

"He broke my heart but not my spirit. NEXT!"

VISUALIZE SUCCESS

It is no secret that Olympic athletes win more medals after they have visualized themselves outperforming their competition and executing their craft to perfection. Visualization also increases your intelligence by boosting the number of interconnectors between the neurons (brain cells) in your brain. It's like "exercising" your brain muscle.

In a study published in the *Journal of Neurophysiology*, Drs. Guang Yue and Kelly Cole had one group of participants exercise a finger for a month while another group just imagined exercising the same finger. Results showed that the group that performed the physical exercise gained strength in the finger by 30 percent, while the imagining group gained finger strength by 22 percent. How astounding is the power of the mind to influence the body.[5]

LAUGH

Can you laugh yourself happy? The answer is yes. Just thinking about having a good laugh is enough to lower stress hormones. According to a Loma Linda University study, researchers told one group of men that they would be watching a funny video and another group was offered magazines to read. The funny video group had much lower levels of stress hormones than the magazine group, *and* the drop in their stress hormones began *before* the film had even begun; just anticipating the laugh was that powerful.[8]

PRACTICE YOGA

People suffering from anxiety and/or depression have low levels of a brain chemical (neurotransmitter) called GABA in their brains. Many antidepressants help by increasing the GABA levels in the brain, but researchers now claim that yoga also increases GABA. According to a Johns Hopkins study, volunteers performing a 1-hour session of yoga twice a week for 4 months increased their GABA levels by 27 percent.[9] As discussed on page 58, yoga has many beneficial consequences for both mind and body. It gets you focused on your breath, triggering the relaxation response, brings bloodflow and release of tension to your muscles, helps calm the mind in a meditative way, and changes brain chemistry.[10] If you cannot make it to a class, there are many audio and visual aids to get you going.

TAKE A COLD SHOWER

According to a recent study published in *Medical Hypotheses*, cold showers have the capacity not only to lift depression but also to possibly prevent it.[11] Hanover Medical School had two groups of participants take either cold or warm showers and found that after 2 to 3 months, the cold shower group had half the number of colds and that their colds were less intense and/or of shorter duration. The Thrombosis Research Institute in London found in their cold-water studies that participants experienced a rise in sex hormones, reduced heart attacks due to improved circulation, increase in white blood cells, harder fingernails, increased hair growth, and "renewed energy." Varicose veins were also positively affected.[12] In another study published in *The Journal of Personality and Social Psychology*, 55 percent of participants reported successful results from water therapy to lower their stress levels and increase their energy.[13]

Wow. Some of the reasoning is that since the skin possesses three to ten times more nerve receptor sites for cold than for warmth, cold water excites the sympathetic nervous system (the one that excites your body), causing your brain to produce that adrenaline drug, which acts as a mild antidepressant. All this stimulation of the nerve cells on your skin has an overwhelming effect, which counteracts depression–sort of like your personal form of electroshock therapy. The authors of the study recommend showering for 2 to 3 minutes in 68°F water twice a day.

I recently got an unplanned cold shower. I walked into my health club and the front desk person told me that the hot water heater was being repaired and she didn't know when it would be up and running. I thought nothing of it and proceeded to perform my 31 minutes of interval strength training, because there was *no* other logical option. After I was done, I forgot about the whole cold water issue and flipped the water on and walked in. My *entire* body jumped when hit with the truly freezing pelts of water. I got out of there fast.

As I was drying off, a few regulars walked by, and I said, "Guys, it's not pretty in there," to which they said smugly, "Oh, we'll be fine." Within moments I heard the screams and yelps of little girls, and they, too, were out drying off in a minute. We laughed that you really don't think it's going to be that bad until you experience it.

The interesting part of the story came two days later, when I saw those same two guys again. I asked, "Ready for another cold shower?" to which they both replied, "You know, it was horrible when it happened, but we both really felt pumped the rest of the day." I thought about it and then realized that I also had a really jazzed day after my cold shower blast. I say give it a try.

CREATE A MENTAL SCREENSAVER

Based on the teachings of Dr. Jeff Zeig, a brilliant psychologist who helps clients get mentally and emotionally unstuck, Cynthia came up with a technique that she calls the Screensaver. We all know how important a screensaver is for the health and well-being of our computer, right? Early monitors could get images literally burned and etched permanently in the screen if left on for too long. I liken these burned images to our early traumatic and embarrassing experiences that are forever embedded in our memories.

We now need to replace those obsolete, burned-in images. Get ready to create your fun, user-friendly, sexy, productive, provocative, adventurous image–the Screensaver. This is your first visualization to usher in hope, faith, and more brain cell connections, which boost intelligence and creative potential.

The most recent client Cynthia taught this technique to was a successful attorney who was divorcing her unemployed husband, who had all the time in the world to spend thousands of *her* dollars buying gifts for *his* girlfriend. In the courtroom, Cynthia's client found it impossible not to engage in verbal legalese battles with her spouse, her spouse's attorney, and even her *own* attorney–after all, she was a brilliant litigator. She was consumed with rage every moment of the day and night–even her dreams were filled with combative courtroom scenarios. As Buddha said, "Holding on to anger is like grasping a hot coal with the intent of throwing it at someone else; you are the one who gets burned." Along the same line, my favorite saying is "Resentment is the poison *you drink* hoping that the other

The Danger of Anger

Research shows that just 5 minutes of recalled anger lowers IgA [the first line of defense against bacteria, which defends our respiratory, gastrointestinal, and urinary tracts from infection] for more than 6 hours. On the other hand, 5 minutes of positive feeling states of care and compassion not only decreased bad mood but also significantly increased IgA levels, which lasted longer than a 6-hour period.[14]

person will die." Think about that for a moment; you resent someone for something and think and/or say horrible things. Who drinks that poison? YOU!

Cynthia's client's anger was actually lowering her antibody production of IgA. She was frequently sick and suffered terrible migraines. When Cynthia asked her client to visualize what image it would take to be able to displace her anger and allow her attorney to do his job, her answer was finally to visualize her spouse and his lawyer sitting on a heap of sh$%&t! The only subsequent problem was that now her client could barely keep from bursting into laughter in the courtroom.

She called her Screensaver "Sh$%&t Happens."

Create your personal Screensaver, and burn it into your mind's hard drive, where it can be brought forward whenever you feel yourself returning to past or future doom and gloom. Replace your anger with your perfect soul-fulfilling image.

How to Create Your Personal Screensaver

It's important to start with a relaxed body, so take a few minutes to use your breathing techniques or meditation. Then grab a piece of paper, take a few deep breaths, fill up your lungs and chest with oxygen, and write down your answers to the following:

1. Start by visualizing a picture of a peaceful and contented you, after you have overcome whatever issue is currently bothering you most.
2. What are you doing in the picture?
3. Where are you?
4. How are you feeling?
5. Is anyone there with you?
6. Give your picture a title. Place it anywhere on your Screensaver and say the title aloud as you focus on your scene.

The Screensaver should be an image that represents how you would like your life to appear and how you feel when it happens. Your image does not have to be realistic and can change over time. Once you perfect your image and can recall it easily, you may develop another Screensaver that concerns another situation in your life that needs alteration or design.

When I did this exercise for myself, my image was seeing *The 7-Day Energy Surge* as #1 on the *New York Times* bestseller list. I'm not kidding or saying this to be funny. I actually see the list, which starts with number one at the top and moves on down. I think about that Screensaver at least a half dozen times each day and simply call it "Go Energy Go!"

This exercise feels great, and by returning often to your desired mental image, you are strengthening its power by shifting and reinforcing new patterns in your brain, while at the same time stimulating your creative resources and moving away from energy-draining obsolete habits.

In addition to these techniques, Cynthia and I came up with the following two exercises as we were trying to effectively purge the mind and body of lethargy and negativity.

MIND-SET EXERCISE 1

Throw It Away

1. Stand with your feet shoulder-width apart. With your arms hanging at your sides, palms up, curl your fingers upward as if you were holding softballs in your hands, and feel the imagined heaviness of your situation, the sadness, anger, and fear. Just hold it and feel it in your hands.

2. Now I want you to turn your palms behind you because you are going to toss this negativity toward the back wall. Swing your arms with force, back and forth, and imagine throwing whatever difficulty you are experiencing behind you. Let momentum do its work. Think of the negativity as sticking to your hands, like drying mud, so you really have to throw and flick it back forcefully to get it off.

3. As you throw your arms back, breathe out; as you swing your arms forward, breathe in. You are getting rich oxygen into your body as you fling the negativity behind you. Feeling a little difference in energy?

4. After a minute or two of swinging your arms like a monkey, you will feel the tightness in your upper body give way, and you'll probably hear a bunch of cracks and pops, so be gentle. I do this until I feel the tendons and ligaments loosen and my breathing deepens.

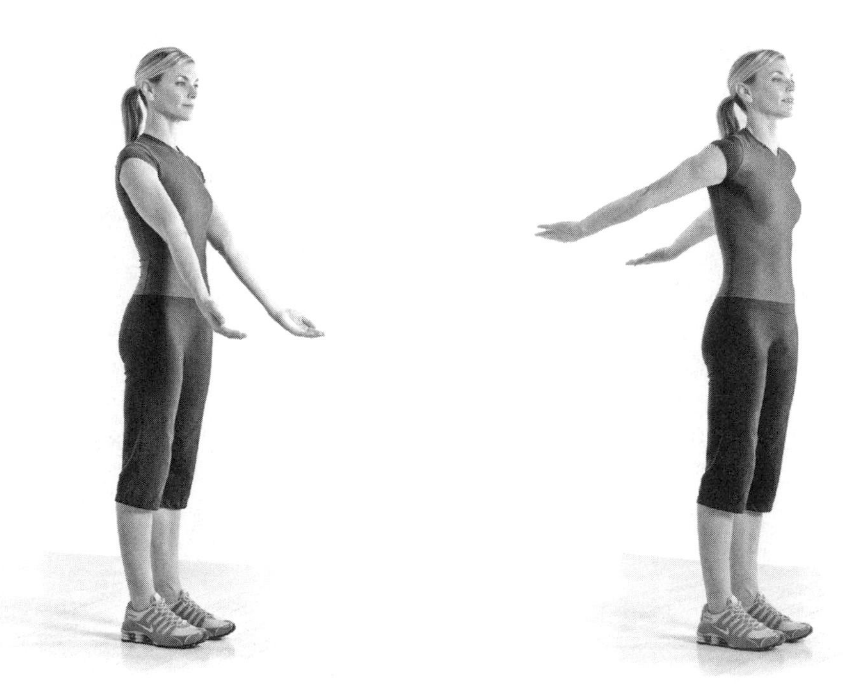

MIND-SET EXERCISE 2

Pat Yourself on the Back

1. Stand with your feet planted on the floor, shoulder-width apart, and think about all the good things you have accomplished throughout your life and what makes you proud.

2. Swing your right arm in front of you and loosely slap the back of your left shoulder with the palm of your right hand. Your hand should be open and limp, not tense or closed.

3. Keep the movement going by now swinging your left arm around to the right side of your body until you slap the back of your right shoulder.

4. With each swing of the arm, turn your head to look behind you, which will loosen all the tension in your neck.

5. Each time you slap yourself on the back, you will hear a thud. Allow that thud to break up tension and tightness.

6. If you are doing this correctly, your arms will fly from right to left with ease and rhythm.

7. Do this for about 2 minutes.

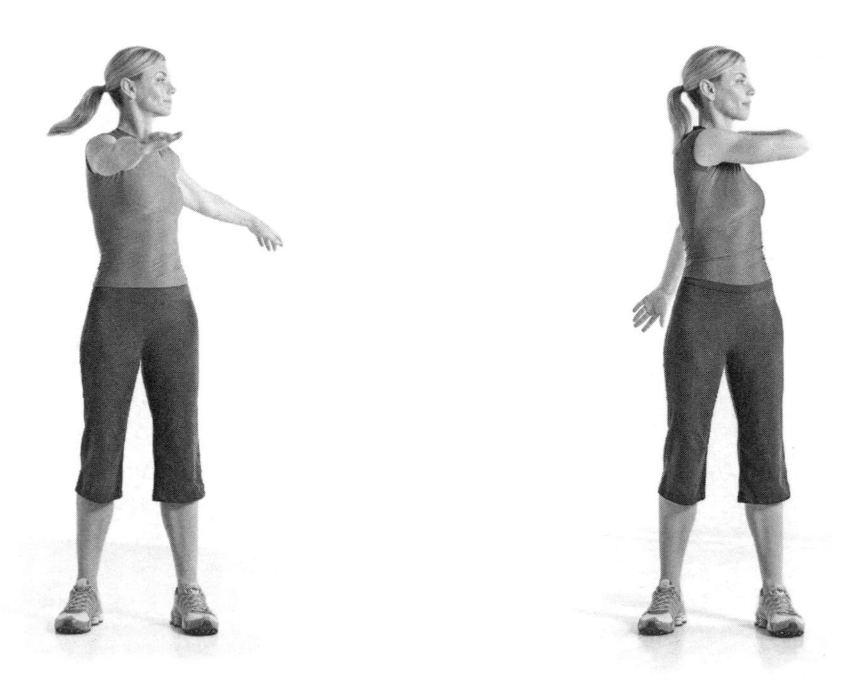

Now that you have awareness of the never-ending communication between the mind and body and the empirical studies demonstrating how they profoundly affect each other, know that your mind-set is of paramount importance to mental health, physical well-being, and the brewing *stew* of energy. Positive, proactive thoughts and behaviors promote and establish long-lasting changes in the brain as well as a steady energetic state.

This component, as well as previous ones, has provided you with many skills to work with your mind/body connection in a healing, rejuvenating manner, using Screensaver, yoga, laughter, Throw It Away, and Pat Yourself on the Back, to name a few.

For this momentous first week, try to monitor several times throughout the day where your mind is drifting and what it is focused on. If you are trapped in the "I must" or "shoulds" or "loser" state of mind, try shifting to the "I would prefers" and "premium thoughts," focusing on what you have learned through your experiences and making more room for possibilities and a more positive state of acceptance. When the shift in language to "I would prefer . . . " is not working, develop and work on your Screensaver image to expand your mind and usher in your creative side. After working with your mind, gently shift to the body movements to free up tension and discomfort. Explore the most efficient and successful ways you can move yourself into a curious, open, welcoming, and optimistic mind-set that will steer your body to a greater sense of strength, vitality, and energy.

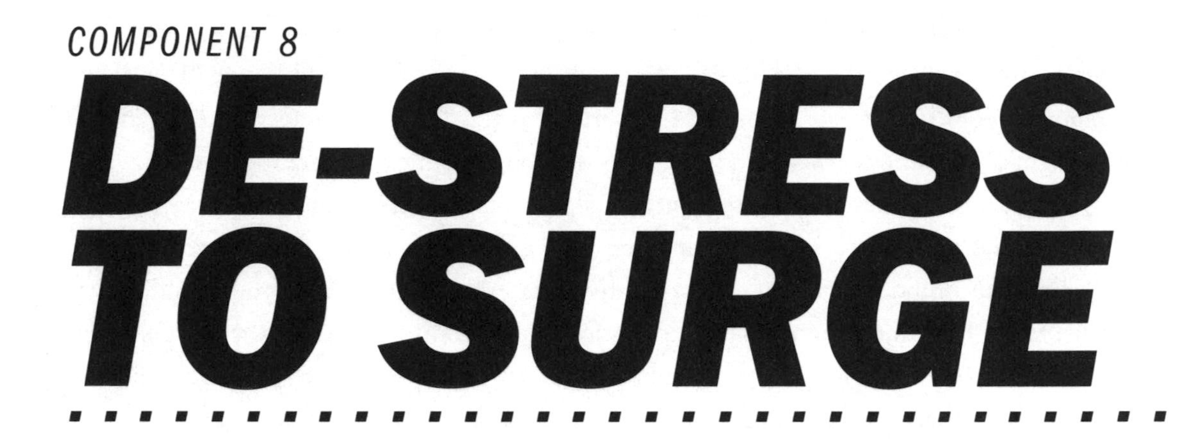
COMPONENT 8
DE-STRESS
TO SURGE

Have you ever walked down a dark hallway only to have someone suddenly appear out of nowhere and scare the living daylights out of you? Can you recall the feeling–heart pounding, accelerated breathing, and ready to run for your life screaming? This reaction is commonly referred to as the "stress response" or the "fight-or-flight" response (which I alluded to earlier in the book), and it's been around for a hundred thousand years; guess we're stuck with it.

THE PROBLEM WITH STRESS

Psychologically speaking, stress is defined as "an imbalance between perceived environmental demands and the individual's perceived resources to cope with these demands."[1] Although it feels like a purely physical experience, the fight-or-flight response includes chemical, physical, and psychological events that prepare us to run like hell, stand and defend ourselves, or even play dead (to survive!).

Our bodies come equipped with special glands that rest on top of the kidneys, called the adrenals; when we are faced with danger, real or perceived, they produce two powerful chemicals of note–adrenaline and cortisol–which move through the bloodstream and cause those reactions that make us want to crawl out of our skin. If you recall, these chemicals are also released when you drink too much coffee or breathe shallowly.

Adrenaline, cortisol, and another stress hormone called norepinephrine bring on the stress response in less than a minute by triggering an increase in blood pressure, heart rate, respiration, tensing of muscles, and increased blood clotting, to name a few, that prepare you for quick action. Although these changes might help you survive a tiger attack, in everyday life, chronic stress robs your body of valuable energy.

Dr. Paul Rosch, president of the American Institute of Stress, claims that "75 to 90 percent of all visits to primary care physicians result from stress-related disorders."[2]

Many studies have been conducted on animals and the consequences of stress. In one study, rats were tied down in a cage and unable to flee, continuously struggling to get free. After repeated exposure to this type of stress, the results showed that the rats were actually gaining weight instead of losing.[3] How was this possible, because they were expending enormous energy struggling to get free *and* not eating?

The answer? During stress our bodies want to conserve energy in order to better fight

CYNTHIA'S CORNER

I work very closely with Beverly Hills–based internist Dr. Soram Khlasa, a pioneer in holistic medicine who was recently elected into the "Best Doctors of America" organization, which was originally affiliated with Harvard University School of Medicine. It was Dr. Khlasa who supported my decision to not do chemotherapy and helped me build my immunity with herbs, supplements, diet, meditation, and yoga. Almost all of Dr. Khlasa's referrals to me concern how stress is wreaking havoc on his patients' state of health. Not all stress is bad; some stress can actually be healthy, because active challenges can stimulate learning, creativity, and a sense of mastery when an individual feels that he/she has some sense of control and influence and sees an effort-reward payoff. But when stress is prolonged and a person perceives that she does not possess the skills to cope with the situation or environment, that is when we must get to work cognitively and physically to bring about periods of rest and rejuvenation for healing, growth, and the retrieval of new or lost resources. There are many things you can do with your mind and body to relieve stress, so keep reading.

or flee. Stress hormones deliver messages not only to release fats, sugar, and insulin into the bloodstream, so we have the energy to flee, but also to store fat and tell the body to eat more. I know that some of my seriously overweight clients fall perfectly into this category.

To add insult to injury, this stress response and its hormonal concoction also slow down your metabolism and shut down digestion, physical growth, reproduction, and the immune system to *save* energy. As a result, we gain weight and wreak havoc on our mind, body, and energy.

To make matters worse, cortisol (there's that nasty bugger again!) directs the body to store fat in the belly–so close to our hearts. Cortisol also bullies leptin, the "good hormone" I introduced you to on page 104 that produces a feeling of fullness. Too much cortisol has also been shown to inhibit the growth of new cells in the part of the brain that controls fear and heightened emotions and forms new memories. Therefore, if you're overly stressed out, you become more easily fearful and forgetful. NOT a good combo.

In two independent studies comparing women who experienced chronic anxiety versus women who didn't, the anxious women had higher levels of bad cholesterol, triglycerides, insulin, and cortisol, and lower levels of thyroid hormone, good cholesterol, and testosterone (which gives you pep and sexual drive, maintains muscle mass, and helps burn fat). And these anxious women had more weight around their bellies.[4] Surprised?

These days, although not regularly confronted by dangerous beasts, we do face the stresses of work, making money, raising children, navigating a relationship, having no relationship, eating toxic foods, not getting enough sleep, being ill, having negative fear-producing thoughts, you name it, life's challenges, which create stress reactions. Like the lab rats, our brains can recall stressful memories; unlike the rats, we fret and worry and have the ability to imagine stresses that have *not* even occurred yet!

When stress is chronic, the feedback loop that is supposed to make the brain tell the adrenals to stop pumping out cortisol becomes faulty and they just keep pumping away. Or the body produces some cortisol but not enough to signal the adrenals to completely stop, therefore preventing recovery in the form of rest, healing, digestion, reproduction, and sleep.

This is similar to what I discussed in Component 2, when you push the pancreas beyond its limits by consuming too much sugary sh$%^t and blow it out. Remember again, the human body is very, very smart, but at times, very, very fragile. Autoimmune disorders and a weakened immune system is the fight-or-flight response in a frenzy.

> *Note:* Recall the previous chapter and the research that just *anticipating* laughter reduced stress hormones. Now, we learn that all we have to do is *anticipate* danger and the physiological fight-or-flight chain of events is off and running. Clearly, anticipation is a powerful state of mind, depending upon where you are going with it.

To be fair to cortisol, it's important to know that natural cortisol production first thing in the morning helps you wake up and energize. Throughout the day, our bodies go through a process called the basic rest-activity cycle (BRAC). It starts with cortisol being produced every 90 to 120 minutes to help you be productive and deal with a changing, demanding environment. About an hour and a half after the cortisol is released, our bodies produce a rest and relaxation chemical called beta-endorphin, which peaks for about 20 minutes.

If you want to get fancy, this 90- to 120-minute period is referred to as an ultradian cycle/rhythm, which means any cycle less than 20 hours, as opposed to the familiar circadian 24-hour cycle that occurs with wake/sleep. So what is important to note here is that after every hour and a half to 2 hours of arousal (physical or mental work), your very smart human body has a built-in mechanism (beta-endorphin) for rest and rejuvenation. Your body will let you know that it is time for a break by yawning, sighing, not concentrating, and feeling fatigued. Step away from the computer and take a 10- to 20-minute break to facilitate and not fight your body's secretion of beta-endorphin for healing. Now, it's not always possible to lie down and close your eyes for a quick nap, but a few minutes of some of the techniques presented below will suffice to respect your body's natural rhythm to maintain health.

STRESS REDUCTION TECHNIQUES

The next time you are stressed out and devoid of energy, do not go along with your habitual inclination to push through, grab some coffee or a sugary snack, and ignore your body's warning sign that it needs a break. Pushing through will ultimately lead to a chronic stress loop, ushering in poor memory and performance, irritability, depression, and illness. Instead, try one of the following stress reduction techniques, which will be incorporated into your 7-day plan.

WATER THERAPY

As mentioned in the previous chapter, don't forget the benefits of water therapy, whether it be a cold shower, a warm bath, a Jacuzzi, or a dip in a swimming pool, lake, or ocean. Water is tremendously effective for calming and soothing your mind and body, and it is known to lower stress levels and increase energy.[5]

EXERCISE

It goes without saying that exercise is a great stress reliever. I call it my "therapy," and when I am feeling stressed out and/or irritable, I perform some of the interval strength-training exercises or just hit the floor and pump out 20+ pushups. Ladies, if the pushups aren't your thing, then try some squats or lunges or simply perform the plank exercise on page 60.

Note: Given the upheaval in our financial markets, my trainers in New York and Chicago are experiencing an increase in business, because many men and women are turning to exercise as the ultimate stress reliever. I couldn't agree with them more.

BREATHING

As discussed in Component 5, Breathe to Surge, working with your breath is truly one of the easiest and most direct ways to alleviate stress. Remember the West Virginia study where just 10 minutes of focused breathing reduced stress up to 44 percent by triggering the relaxation response?[6, 7] Go back and review the techniques of Breathing into Blackness, Alternate-Nostril Breathing, and Breath of Fire.

TEA TIME

According to University College of London, drinking four cups of black tea a day lowered cortisol, reduced the risk of heart attacks, and promoted relaxation after a stressful task.[8]

CHEWING GUM

Australian researchers found that gum chewing helps relieve tension. Those who chewed gum during math and memory tests experienced a 17 percent decrease in self-reported stress. The author of the study, Andrew Scholey, said that the "act of chewing may subconsciously be associated with positive social settings like mealtimes and this association may reduce stress."[9] Interesting.

MEDITATION

The goal of meditation is to carve out a peaceful chunk of time where the brain or mind is not attached or engaged in thoughts of the past or future, but just being in the moment with an awareness for when thoughts arise.

The additional benefits of a few minutes of meditation each day include:[10, 11]

- Lowered respiration and heart rate
- Decreased muscular tension
- Increased alpha (relaxing) brain waves
- Reduced oxygen consumption
- Alteration in the structure of the brain that deals with attention, sensory processing, and happiness

Blue Cross–Blue Shield did a study tracking 2,000 meditators and found them to be much healthier with regard to physical and mental diseases, especially heart disease (an 87 percent reduction compared to those who didn't meditate).[12, 13]

Still not convinced? A study from England also found that for each year that you meditate, you can take off one year of aging.[14]

I witnessed the power of meditation firsthand. A few years back, I worked with Hugh Jackman while he was starring in *The Boy from Oz* on Broadway, for which he won a Tony Award. Hugh *never* missed a performance (I take that back, he had to cancel one show because he hosted the Tony Awards–talk about stressful!), including previews and a run that lasted more than 14 months. The show was more than 2½ hours long, had eight performances a week, and is believed to be the single most demanding starring role ever written in a musical, as it required Hugh to perform 20 songs. What did he do to accomplish this task? He:

- Ate right
- Drank tons of water
- Avoided almost all alcohol
- Slept a minimum of 8 hours a night and frequently took short naps
- Exercised (with me) three times a week
- MEDITATED for a total of 1 to 2 hours each and every day

To this day, Hugh continues to get it all right. I just returned from 3 weeks of training him in Vancouver, where he is finishing up his next movie, *X-Men Origins: Wolverine,* which will release in May 2009. At this point, he is juggling filming, preparing to host the Academy Awards, producing and planning his next movie/theater vehicle, moving into a new home, and being a very present husband and father. Where does Hugh get the energy? He keeps doing many of the things I'm urging you to do, all outlined in this book (most of which he figured out on his own, and some he actually taught me).

Physiologist Dr. Robert Keith Wallace spent decades studying the effects of meditation on health and found that meditators who had practiced for more than 5 years were biologically 12 years younger than their chronological age when compared with those who did not meditate. The meditators had better blood pressure, vision, and hearing. Short-term meditators were about 5 years younger than their chronological age, so it's never too late to start.[15, 16]

The part of the brain responsible for positive states such as joy, happiness, and compassion (left frontal lobe) showed increased activity in the brain scans of meditators versus nonmeditators. And after 4 months, meditators still reported significant reductions in anxiety as well as increased positive feelings.[17]

A Word from Our Testers

"I find the meditation/de-stress exercises easier if I pretend I am in a different place. Visual aids may help, too."
—*Marsha M., age 56*

Another benefit of meditation is that your eyes move from sharp focus to soft focus, as I urged you to do when you get up in the middle of the night. Sharp focus, also known as tunnel vision, is part of the stress response as an animal locks its eyes on its predator. When the eyes are locked for any length of time–on a computer, television, video game, or reading–the muscles of the eyes, neck, and face tense up and diaphragmatic breathing decreases. So every hour or so, look away from what you are doing, stare at the sky or at water, or close your eyes and gently massage them with your fingertips; this might even be a good time to visualize your feel-good Screensaver. Remember all that stuff about your breath? When you soften your focus, your facial muscles relax, and that signals the body to follow suit; it also helps to smile. According to brain scientists, soft focus decreases the stress response and moves your brain from linear, left-brain mode to the holistic and creative right-brain mode.

TAPPING

I am a firm believer that when you work with your mind you cannot ignore your body. At the end of this chapter, you'll find a simple, healing, antistress technique that Cynthia taught me. It has been around for more than 20 years and was developed by George Goodheart, Dr. Roger J. Callahan, and Gary Craig. It deals with the mind and body at the same time and is based on the fundamentals of chakras and meridians, similar to acupuncture.

We all know our bodies have an electrical system and energy fields. Meridians are energy pathways, which carry the flow of energy from the top of our head to the bottom of our toes and from muscles to organs. Modern researchers have documented the existence of meridians using radioactive isotopes and imaging–something Chinese physicians discovered more than 5,000 years ago. Eastern medicine believes that trauma, stress, and emotional wounds from our past can cause blockages in these energy highways. These blockages disrupt our body's energy flow, thus causing mental and physical lethargy and illness.

When an acupuncturist inserts a tiny needle into a specific point on your body's energy pathway, this stimulation helps release the blockage and get the energy flowing, "sending electrochemical impulses to your brain and releasing neurotransmitters."[18] Once again, neurotransmitters are brain chemicals that move information throughout your brain and body.

Back in 1997, even the U.S. National Institutes of Health claimed that "the data in support of acupuncture are as strong as those for many accepted Western medical therapies."[19] This same report also stated that acupuncture caused the body to release hormones (peptides) that resemble opium, which explains why acupuncture has been effective in relieving physical pain and discomfort.

The beauty of this technique is that we will *not* be using needles–just our fingers–to activate specific acupuncture points and stimulate the flow of blood, lymph, and energy. This tapping technique has many names, including "thought field therapy," "the emotional freedom technique," and "meridian therapy." It is very similar to acupressure in that you are physically touching your body, but it is different in that you are also including your mental state at the same time by thinking about what is disturbing you. Many people find great benefits from acupressure, but this goes one step further in recognizing once again the mind/body connection.

Although controversial, these techniques have been shown by some to create positive results for people with heart irregularities by improving heart rate variability. Remember that enhancing heart rate variability is the reason why you are strength-training in intervals.[20] Convinced you need to tap yet?

ACUPRESSURE

Acupressure is derived from acupuncture, where physical pressure is placed on certain points on the body using hands, elbows, and certain devices. Although many find it therapeutic, there aren't currently well-conducted clinical studies to back up its effectiveness, but researchers are beginning to study it more. According to an article in the *American Journal of Nursing*, many states are training nurses in this type of therapy. The article goes on to mention the benefits of meridian therapy (acupressure) for treating pain and nausea, increasing immunity and relaxation, and decreasing blood pressure and withdrawal symptoms of addiction.[21] If you cannot find or afford a knowledgeable meridian or acupressure therapist, there are many books and maps of the human body that show you where to press for what malady.

FELDENKRAIS®

The Feldenkrais Method® accesses our ability to learn or relearn how to move with greater efficiency. A Feldenkrais "lesson" consists of gentle, precise movements that develop and direct our awareness of how we do what we do. Each "lesson," and there are hundreds with infinite variety, addresses some function such as sitting, standing, jumping, rolling. The benefits are improved balance, coordination, ease and well-being. The two modalities of the Feldenkrais Method are verbally instructed lessons in a group class and private hands-on lessons lying fully clothed on a padded Feldenkrais table. I first was exposed to it at Studio C in Beverly Hills with Claire Nettle. As I lay on the massage table, she gently tugged and nudged all areas of my body from my toes to my ears. Throughout the session I kept yawning and feeling my body sink deeply into the table. All tension left my body and when I got up, I found myself standing taller with an open chest, as if my spinal column had realigned itself. My head felt lighter and as if it had moved back a few inches and was now perfectly poised between my shoulders as I floated out of the studio. I truly recommend this experience.

EYE MOVEMENT DESENSITIZATION AND REPROCESSING

A protocol developed by Dr. Francine Shapiro, eye movement desensitization and reprocessing (EMDR) is based on the fact that when the left and right hemispheres of the brain are stimulated bilaterally, which involves any movement, sound, or touch that goes back and forth from right to left or left to right, coping skills are more accessible.

Dr. Shapiro worked with Vietnam War veterans and found that when they recalled traumatic memories and located where they felt tension in their bodies, and moved their eyes from side to side, amazing results occurred.

A study funded by Kaiser Permanente showed that 100 percent of single-trauma and 80 percent of multiple-trauma survivors were no longer diagnosed with post-traumatic stress disorder (PTSD) after six 50-minute sessions.[22] That is an astounding benefit in only 300 total minutes. Anyone suffering from PTSD should go to www.emdr.com and click on "Find an EMDR Clinician."

You cannot do EMDR on yourself, but Cynthia and I have found that when upset, if we focus on our breathing and body, and do some sort of touching or movement that goes from right to left (such as tapping on your outer thighs or shoulders), the stress usually dissipates and oftentimes disappears.

LISTENING TO MUSIC

The latest research on the effects of music and the relaxation response is overwhelming. Music is so important to your well-being that I have devoted an entire component to it. Just know that in regard to stress, scientists believe that listening to peaceful music may inhibit the release of the adrenal stress hormones when your body goes into that fight-or-flight mode.[23] According to Dr. Daniel Levitin at McGill University in Montreal and author of *This Is Your Brain on Music*, music arouses your brain's pleasure centers, which may help lower blood pressure; improve quality of sleep; and alleviate pain, depression, and anxiety.[24]

Note: You might want to drink tea as you listen to music to hit a solid "double" for your energy.

Now here are a few simple exercises that will help you put these techniques into action.

DE-STRESS EXERCISE 1

Meditation

Here is a form of meditation from Thich Nhat Hanh, a well-known Vietnamese monk and peace activist. He currently resides in France because he was banned from his country for helping war refugees and espousing peace. He has written numerous books about mindfulness, meditation, and inner and world peace. The meditation below is his simple technique to bring about "oneness of body and mind."

1. Soften your eyes by gazing downward, about 2 to 3 feet in front of you, or if you prefer, close them.
2. Take a few deep breaths, and with each inhalation silently say to yourself, "I know that I am breathing in."
3. With each exhalation, say to yourself, "I know that I am breathing out."

If you are doing this with some degree of awareness, you will not be able to have any other thoughts, because there is no way you can keep track of your "in and out breaths" and pair them with the above phrases if you are thinking about something else. Try it for a few minutes and draw your own conclusions. If you do get off track and find yourself engaging in thought, don't get mad or frustrated and declare, "I just can't meditate!" Instead, just label the thought, "Thinking," and go back to the in breath with "I know that I am breathing in," followed by the out breath, "I know that I am breathing out." Try this for 2 to 3 minutes and build up to 10 to 20 minutes.

DE-STRESS EXERCISE 2

Tapping to Happy

Cynthia and I developed our own tapping recipe. We call it, "Tapping to Happy." It only takes a few minutes and will help you heal your heart and soul.

1. Think about what is stressing you out—a memory, situation, feeling, or behavior—and give it a detailed name, such as "Anger toward my spouse," "Pain in my back," or "Difficulty at work."

2. On a scale of 0 to 10, where 0 is no disturbance and 10 is about as bad as it gets, give this stressor a number and write it down.

3. With the index, third, and ring fingers of your dominant hand, using a small circular motion, firmly massage your upper chest on the side opposite your dominant hand (e.g., use your right hand to massage your upper left chest or vice versa), starting just below your collarbone and moving directly under the bone toward the area where your collarbone meets your shoulder bone. You should feel some areas of soreness, which indicate where congestion is occurring. When you find an especially sore spot, massage it firmly and say aloud the following statements:

   - "Even though I struggle with this (insert name of issue), I completely and deeply accept myself."
   - "Even though I struggle with this (insert name of issue), I completely and deeply respect myself."
   - "Even though I struggle with this (insert name of issue), I completely and deeply love myself."

4. Now firmly tap where your eyebrow starts (the side near your nose and just above the bridge). Tap firmly about 20 times per location. Keep thinking about your issue throughout your tapping.

5. Tap the outer corner of the same eyebrow, on the bony ridge above the eye socket. Again, repeat to yourself the name of your issue.

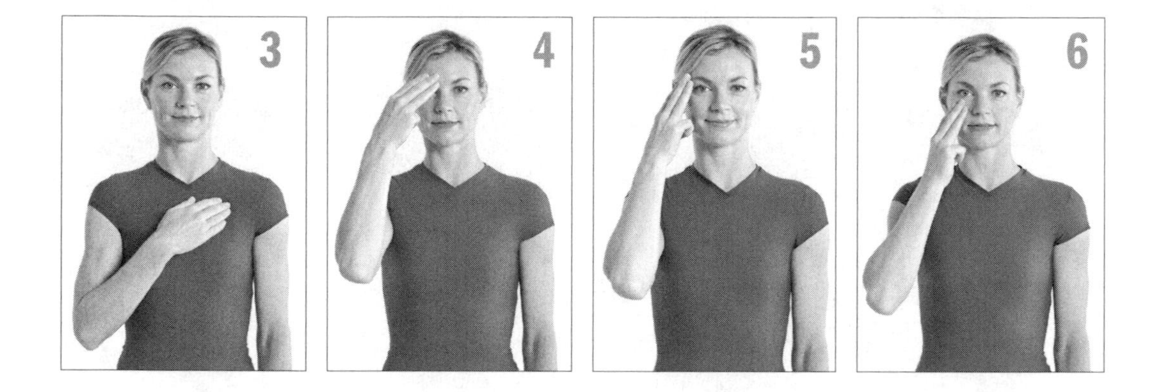

6. Tap on the bone right under the middle of the same eye, just above your cheekbone.

7. Tap right under your nose, just above your upper lip.

8. Tap the middle of your chin.

9. Tap your chest under one of your collarbones, about 1 inch below and 1 inch from the middle of your chest over toward your arm.

10. Tap the middle of your sternum.

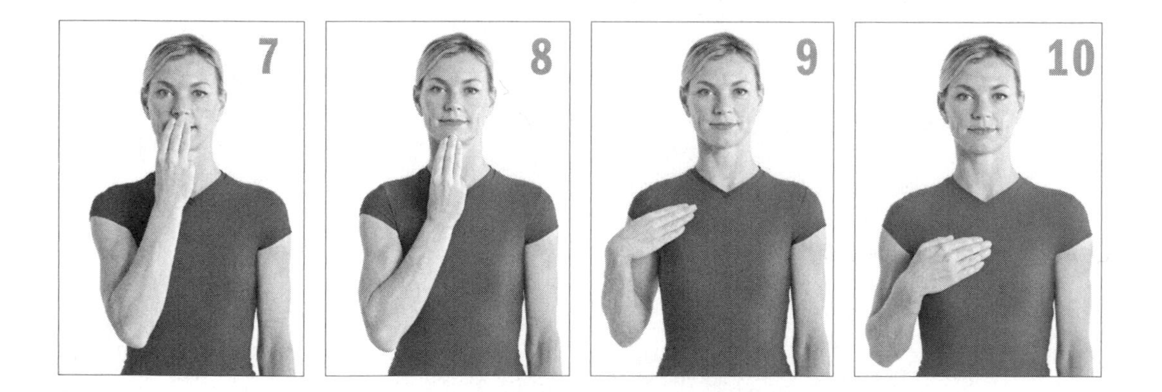

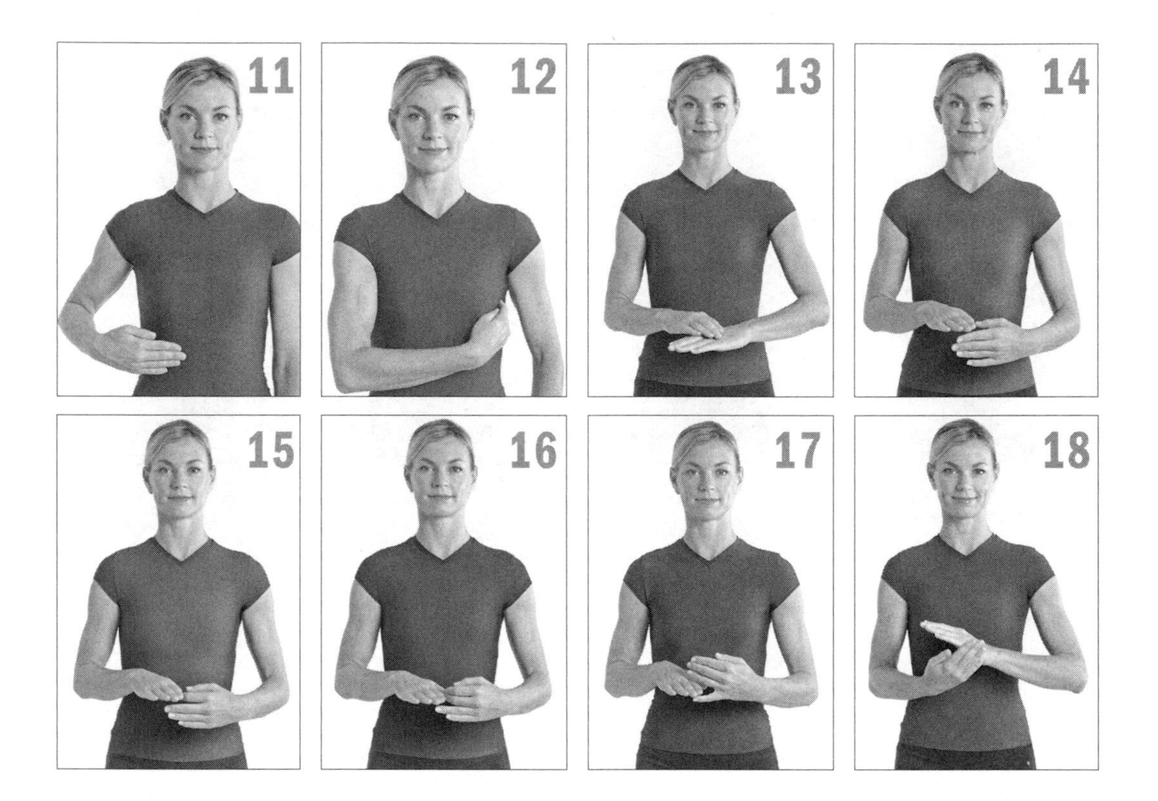

11. Tap 3 inches below your nipple on your rib cage.

12. Tap under your opposite arm, 4 inches below your armpit.

13. Tap the top of your hand between the tendons of the fourth and fifth fingers.

14. Tap the side of your index finger (the one closest to the thumb) where the nail begins.

15. Tap the side of your middle finger where the nail begins.

16. Tap the side of your fourth finger where the nail begins.

17. Tap the side of your pinky where the nail begins.

18. Tap the outer edge of your hand, the area between the wrist and knuckle (the part you would use to karate chop).

Take a deep breath and, once again, rate your disturbance when you think of your issue, and write the new number down next to the old one. If the number is the same or still high, perform another round or two of the tapping.

Note: If you find that a specific location feels especially good, tap longer; this clearly represents an energy block that needs to be opened and requires more time.

DE-STRESS EXERCISE 3

Picking Apples in the Sky

When Cynthia was a little girl, her family would go apple picking on a farm bordering Illinois and Wisconsin. The cool, fresh air, the warmth of the sun, the smell and taste of the sweet red apples, and the act of stretching up to the sky to pick them combined to create a wonderfully de-stressing multisensory experience, upon which this exercise is based.

1. Start by scanning your body for any sign of tension or tightness and take two deep breaths. Ask yourself, "What's bothering me that is causing this tension?"

2. With your eyes open, visualize yourself standing in your idyllic apple orchard.

3. Stand tall—feet shoulder-width apart. Begin to inhale and with your right hand reach upward and really stretch toward the sky to pick an apple. It's higher than you thought; so exaggerate the reach, look upward, and grab your imaginary apple.

4. As you bring your apple down, exhale slowly and deeply and allow your hand to hang at your side.

5. Now reach for the sky and pick an apple with your left hand—breathing in the entire time—and once again, grab your apple and start to lower your left arm while exhaling.

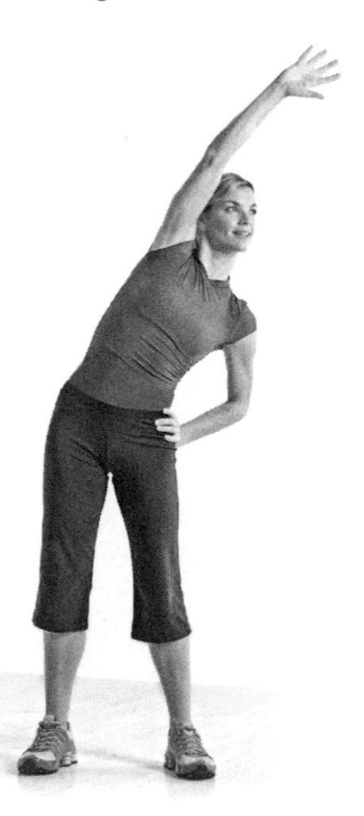

6. With each reach for an apple, make that apple symbolic of what you would like to attain. For example, when you grab your apple, you can say to yourself, "Here is my apple for health . . . wealth . . . love . . ." Say anything you'd like to achieve or have.

7. Do this for 2 to 3 minutes, until you have established a nice rhythm, a stretch that feels good, and a mind/body connection to something you wish to attain.

Aside from getting a nice spinal, arm, and shoulder stretch, you are oxygenating your body (we talked about this in Component 5), disengaging from thought, and bilaterally stimulating your brain.

Now you should have more awareness for where your mind wanders, obsesses, and stresses. You can start to guide it toward a more positive, open, and optimistic point of view with the new skills and resources presented in this component and the preceding one on mindset. But we all know how life can and will slam us with sudden and unexpected events, sending our stress levels soaring and hindering our health and energy if prolonged.

At times we may feel overwhelmed and unable to control our anxiety, fear, or physical reactions to this stress. But there are things you can do to be proactive in small but powerful ways. Do not forget to respect your body's basic rest/activity cycles throughout the day, and take those necessary breaks when your body tells you it's tired and your mind cannot focus. Use laughter, breathing, and meditation to calm your anxious nervous system, and then incorporate physical movement, such as yoga, exercise, Tapping to Happy, and Picking Apples in the Sky, to help your mind/body discharge the toxins and negativities.

Remember: Stress Down = Energy UP!

COMPONENT 9

MUSIC APPRECIATION 101 TO SURGE

When was the last time you were driving and a great song came on the radio? Did you crank up the volume and start to sing along, even if you sounded like Rosanne Barr butchering the national anthem? Wasn't it fun, and weren't you instantly jazzed?

Quick–what's your favorite song? I know it might be embarrassing, but you know that it always lifts your spirits, even if it's "Feelings." Remember the last party or wedding you attended, perhaps feeling sorry for yourself for being single, or worse yet, wishing you were there–single? Have you ever had a fight with your date only to hear some great tune, causing you to sing, dance, and eventually forget what the argument was all about?

That's how powerful music can be to our mind, body, spirit, and ENERGY, and the research is compelling and unanimous. In the past two decades, new brain-imaging techniques have linked music and its effects on our nervous system to improved mood and well-being. Mental, emotional, and physical energy gets a big boost every time you immerse yourself in an ocean of music that moves you.

I play music EVERYWHERE: in my home, office, and car, and am virtually inconsolable when I realize that I have forgotten my iPod and am about to work out. I know for a fact that I have inspired my family, friends, and co-workers to do the same, and I notice more and more of them playing music in all different settings and they seem to be happier and snappier.

Music is a multifaceted auditory stimulus of rhythm, melody, tempo, pitch, form, timbre, and style. Whether you play an instrument or just listen, here is what happens when we listen to music:

- The outer ear captures the vibrations and patterns
- Then sends it to the middle ear to amplify
- Then passes the sound to the inner ear
- Where it changes the mechanical energy of these vibrations into electrical energy
- Which is then transmitted to the brain

What then happens is that the brain reacts to the sound by shifting our focus, releasing hormones, and activating emotions and memory. The positive and relaxing effect that music has on our brain cells and hormones brings about an increase in our healing, immunity, and cellular regeneration.[1, 2, 3]

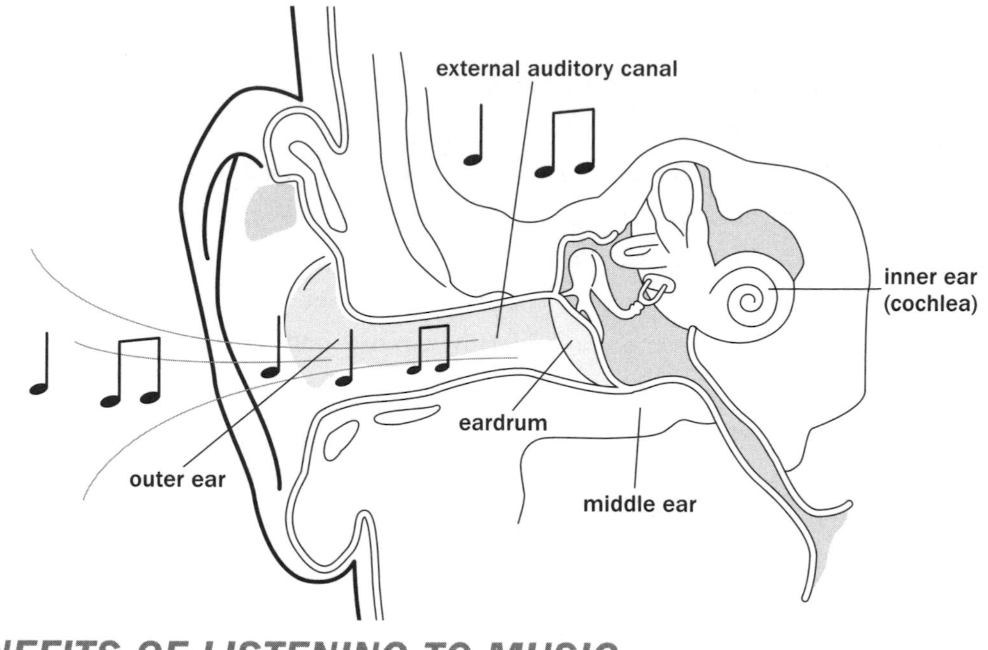

BENEFITS OF LISTENING TO MUSIC

MUSIC UP = DEPRESSION DOWN

Whether it's blasting in your home, car, or iPod, or you are attending a concert for that total sensory immersion, the benefits of listening to music are abundant. In a recent literature review, four out of five studies showed that music therapy was more effective in lifting depression than any other form of therapy. Many studies confirm that music lifts depression; enhances sleep; reduces anxiety, blood pressure, heart rate, stress hormones, and pain; boosts immunity; improves focus and IQ; aids weight loss; promotes healing; and, most important, *energizes*.[4]

Concert, Anyone?

When you go to a concert, symphony, jazz club, or any venue that has live music, you are not only gaining the relaxation and healing response of music but also engaging in other sensory experiences that create novelty and thus stimulation of new brain cells. The vibration of the music stimulates your body, the sight of the band and lights stimulates the visual cortex of your brain, and the hopefully good connection to others creates bonding and togetherness feelings.

CYNTHIA'S CORNER

In my practice, I use music for both depression and anxiety. Music is especially useful to soothe and uplift someone who has just recalled and worked through a past trauma. My clients and I are constantly surprised when the client dips back into a painful past, feels it, mourns it, cries or sobs for almost an hour, then after listening to merely 3 to 5 minutes of beautiful and uplifting music, departs my office feeling both calm and energized. I choose music with melody and lyrics designed to soothe your "inner child," as well as music that is recorded to move from right speaker to left speaker for that added benefit of bilateral stimulation (EMDR) that we spoke about earlier. Note: *Try to use music that has a tempo between 60 and 70 beats per minute, which is about that of a healthy heart rate, to help with anxiety. The volume should also be comfortable. If you are skeptical about getting hooked up to music, famed author Dr. Stephen Levine, a trauma specialist known for his teachings on death and dying, claims that simply recalling a tune and humming it or singing out loud can become an internal resource that soothes you.*

Fifty-six depressed subjects listened to Beethoven's third and fifth piano sonatas for 15 minutes twice a week and as a result their depression, as measured on the standard Beck Depression Scale, decreased.[5]

MUSIC UP = ANXIETY DOWN

In a study at Baltimore Hospital, heart patients derived the same benefits from listening to 30 minutes of music as did those who received 10 milligrams of an antianxiety medication.[6]

MUSIC UP = PAIN DOWN

Looking to reduce pain, anxiety, and stress without medication and its side effects? Reggae musician Bob Marley was way before his time when he said, "One good thing about music–when it hits you, you feel no pain," and these days, when it comes to pain, many experts believe that the relaxing effects of music provide a competing stimulus for those nerve impulses that travel up the spinal column and to the brain, so fewer pain impulses reach your awareness.[7]

Harvard surgeon Dr. Claudius Conrad went along with this program as he played Mozart for his intensive care patients in pain and was amazed to find that they:

Let's Make Music

Making music is not only enjoyable but also has the ability to alleviate stressful mental and physical conditions. The latest findings reveal that playing an instrument or singing is therapeutic. Those playing a musical instrument had a greater reversal of stress hormones after a music lesson than the group that read magazines and newspapers.[8]

Singing in a choral group was also found to benefit both physical and emotional health. In one study, those who sang in a chorus actually boosted their immunity and increased their feelings of well-being.[9] The wonderful thing about singing is that you can join a group or do it solo.

- Needed half as much pain medication as patients who didn't listen
- Had increases in pituitary growth hormone levels, responsible for healing
- Experienced a 20 percent decrease in two known stress hormones.[10]

Men hospitalized with back pain who listened to music for 25 minutes a day slept better and had less pain than men who didn't listen to music.[11, 12] And a 2005 study published in the *European Journal of Anesthesiology* showed that patients who listened to music after hernia surgery required less morphine.[13]

MUSIC UP = BLOOD PRESSURE DOWN

At the University of California at San Diego, researchers stressed participants by giving them a task, then nudging them to go faster. Afterward, the participants listened to different types of music or to silence.[14] The results were:

- Those who did not listen to music had a blood pressure spike of 11 points.
- Jazz and pop listeners had less of a spike.
- Classical music listeners spiked only 2 points.

MUSIC UP = SLEEP UP

At the Sleep Disorders Center in Ohio, Dr. Donna Arand prescribes routine relaxing music at bedtime to signal and condition the body to slow down and get ready for la-la land. In agreement with this finding, a Case Western University study found that listening to easy music for 45 minutes before bedtime slowed breath rate, promoted drifting off to sleep faster, and facilitated a deeper sleep, something I mentioned in Component 6.[15]

In one study, 50 high school students listened to "peaceful music" every night before bedtime for 1 month and 74 percent of these students were able to fall asleep within 10 minutes. In addition, they reported a decrease in nightmares as well as feeling better the next morning and into the day.[16]

MUSIC UP = MEMORY AND ATTENTION UP

In Finland, 60 stroke patients were divided up into those who listened to music and those who did not. The music group had better recovery of memory and better attention skills as well as a more positive outlook. After 3 months, verbal memory improved by 60 percent in the music group.[17]

MUSIC UP = PERFORMANCE UP

When preparing for a speech, an oral presentation, or a review, listen to music, especially Pachelbel's Canon in D. According to an Australian study, listening to Pachelbel prevented stress reactions, such as elevated blood pressure, heart rate, and cortisol levels. Those who didn't listen to music had significant increases in all of these variables.[18]

Children given music lessons as opposed to drama lessons improved their IQ scores by two or three points.[19]

Music and Meals

However, music may not be your friend when it comes to eating and drinking less. Research indicates that fast-paced music stimulates most people to eat and drink more. We know from Components 1, 2, and 3 that our body weight and what we eat and drink has a significant effect on energy. If slow-paced music calms you, by all means play it during meals; a University of Rhode Island study found that people who took their time eating ate 70 fewer calories per meal than those who didn't. If you figure 70 fewer calories, three times a day, that's about a 20-pound weight loss per year![20]

The University of California found that students who listened to 10 minutes of Mozart prior to taking SAT tests had higher scores.[21, 22]

Find yourself struggling through those last few, difficult reps when strength-training? Well, a UK study at York St. John University found that listening to music while holding a 2.4-pound dumbbell straight out in front of the body enabled participants to hold it 10 percent longer than those who opted for white noise or part-time listening. The researchers found that the key to success was what music you selected, especially if it had lyrics that rev you up.[23]

MUSIC = THE ULTIMATE HOSPITAL HELPER

As health care is getting slashed, hospitals are experimenting with the benefits of music by playing live music for preoperative patients as well as children. At Florida State Uni-

Shall We Dance?

The wonderful thing about dance is that it is not only a physical activity but also a comprehensive mind/body experience. Dance is hot these days as a result of the overwhelming success of *Dancing with the Stars,* and dance class participation is on an upswing. The overwhelming benefits of dance include:

- **Calorie burn.** Yes, you do burn a good number of calories, because dancing is different than how you generally use your body. I also like that it involves multiplane movements, similar to the ones in this book's exercise program.
- **Muscle activation.** Core muscles are used as well as ones you never knew you had.
- **Reduced risk of dementia for the elderly,** according to the *New England Journal of Medicine.*[24]
- **Increased bloodflow to the brain.** I hope you realize by now this is *only* energy positive.
- **Mental workout.** You'll need to stay alert as you memorize the steps or keep from stepping on your partner's toes.
- **Decreased stress, depression, and feelings of isolation** because it is frequently a social activity, but feel free to hit the dance floor at home. And for some who dance like Elaine in *Seinfeld,* doing it solo may alleviate some embarrassment.[25]

versity, Jayne Standley found that premature babies breathed better and gained weight more quickly after listening to music.[26, 27] Premies that experienced live music came home 12 days earlier than those who didn't get the music, saving an estimated $2,000 a day.[28]

WHAT MUSIC TO CHOOSE

If the music is familiar and pleasant to you, motor responses arise and you might find yourself doing a Tom Cruise from *Risky Business* or grooving in your car as onlookers chuckle (who cares!).

Just remember to pick your music according to what mental or physical state you'd like to achieve: "Exciting music leads to increased arousal, calming music the reverse."[29] Switch on that upbeat music to awaken, exercise, and recharge, then listen to mellow-mood tunes to relax, eat less, eat *slowly,* stretch out your muscles, or sleep.

To really gain access to the relaxation response, music therapists recommend listening for 20 to 30 minutes. In most instances, the positive effects of music were long lasting and continued even after the subjects stopped listening.

From here on, get up and turn on some music. If you are not a music aficionado and don't know where to start, use the scan button on your radio and pay attention to what perks you up. Find a great music store or bookstore that has easy access to earphones for sampling. If you have ever dreamed of playing a musical instrument, now is the time to get started, and you can borrow, rent, or buy inexpensive used instruments everywhere these days. Purchase concert or symphony tickets, or attend one of the many free musical venues at the parks, churches, museums, restaurants, or bars in your area.

If that seems too daunting, start using your own special vocal instrument and sing, sing, sing. Sing along with your favorite CDs, the radio, commercials, and TV theme songs. Back in the day, mine was *Gilligan's Island*—"Just sit right back and you'll hear a tale . . ."

Music is a tried-and-true bona fide road to increased health, immunity, relaxation, excitation, and "good, good, good, good vibrations," so rock on with classical, country, disco, jazz, house, Latin, hip-hop, or rap—any music that speaks to your soul.

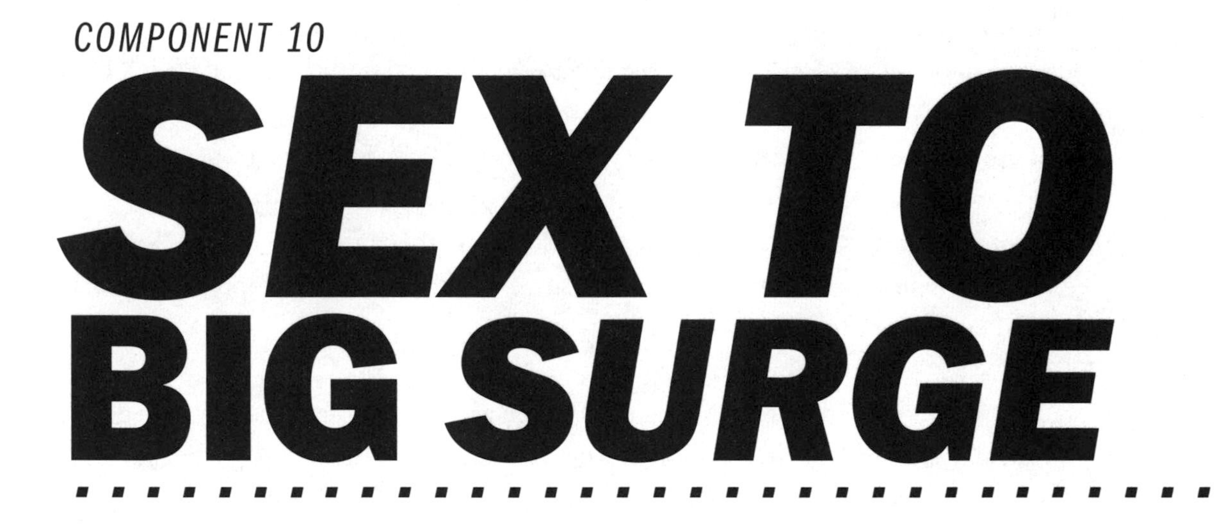
COMPONENT 10
SEX TO
BIG SURGE

Remember the last time you had mind-blowing sex? What was it that enabled you to spend a part of the night (or the entire night, if you were lucky) barely sleeping? What was it that stirred in your mind and body that felt so exhilarating and calming at the same time? Can you recall spending hours exploring another person's body, delighting in so many delicious sensations, basking in the afterglow? Isn't this the energy that we all seek and deserve, and WOW, how great do we feel the following morning and into the next day?

Note: If you are in between mates, don't think you should skip this chapter! There is a lot you can accomplish on your own, and we will get into the prescriptions for "singlehood" in a moment. Don't forget that loving yourself is a prerequisite to being able to receive love as well as love another.

SEXUAL CHEMISTRY 101

What we aren't aware of is the fact that desire and lust are chemical reactions to an exotic "cocktail" of hormones that our bodies produce during the early stages of romantic love; it's this cocktail that stimulates neurons in our brains and just makes us crazy. Unfortunately, this cocktail is a limited onetime shot, and its high only lasts a short while; sorry, no saddling up to the bar and ordering a second round. The evolutionary theory is that these lusty hormones serve to keep us interested long enough for the completion of the biological urge to reproduce, and then they fade once offspring arrive, because how can we tend to our young if we can't leave the bedroom? Not great for species survival.

Michael Liebowitz at New York State Psychiatric Institute blames "crazy love" on two neurotransmitters, or brain chemicals, that communicate information throughout the brain and body:[1]

- **PEA,** which acts like an amphetamine (speed). Mice and monkeys injected with phenylethylamine (PEA) displayed courting gestures and frolicking, fun-loving behavior. (Where can I buy some????)
- **Dopamine,** the euphoric drug also stimulated by coffee and chocolate, causes feelings of ecstasy, creativity, and spontaneity, and the intense ability to focus on another person and further drive up our level of testosterone, consequently boosting our lust and longing.

CYNTHIA'S CORNER

We females have added pheromones called copulins, secreted in the vagina. Pheromones are "a chemical that triggers a natural behavioral response in another member of the same species."[2] During ovulation, copulins are at their highest concentration. When men get a whiff of this fatty acid, it can drive their testosterone levels up by as much as 150 percent and can cause them to find women more desirable.[3] If your man isn't showing enough interest, place his head on your lap and massage his scalp.

Testosterone is produced in the testes and adrenals of men and in the ovaries and adrenals in women. Remember from the exercise chapter that, on average, men produce 40 to 60 times more testosterone than women do, but women are more sensitive to the hormone. This easily explains the gender differences in sexual preoccupation, sex drive, and aggression.[4] For both sexes, sad to say, testosterone declines with age, but with regular sex (that's good), levels do go up (that's better), so go for it (every chance you get). Works for me!

Oscar Wilde once said, "The essence of romance is uncertainty," and there is proof of this in chemistry; when our desire (reward) is thwarted or delayed, like when your hot date doesn't call (or call back) the morning after the first night of lovemaking, our brain cells produce more dopamine, which, in turn, energizes the brain to concentrate and push even harder to attain the "reward"–the love from another person.[5] Playing "hard to get" can be a productive strategy to fuel those obsessive love chemicals in the early stages of a relationship.[6] I am not encouraging game playing, but for some of us, the courtship, quest, and conquering can be a fun and exhilarating ride in life. If it's not your thing (I hate it, but Cynthia lives for the strategy of the kill), follow your own instincts.

Italian scientists have discovered yet another lust hormone, neutrophins, in the bloodstreams of newly intimate men and women.[7] Sadly, a year or two later, this hormone was almost nonexistent in these same couples. Don't be dismayed, though, because they now possessed increased levels of oxytocin, also known as the "cuddle hormone," which makes us feel loved and in need of "warmth and togetherness"; it probably helps mothers bond with their infants, too. Oxytocin also induces milk production and contractions in new and pregnant mothers. In both sexes, oxytocin is released during the act of intercourse and heavy petting. Unfortunately, oxytocin also suppresses testosterone, which might explain waning sexual drive and desire with time. Men release a secondary hormone during sex, called vasopressin, which causes feelings of deep attachment . . . well, maybe.[8]

Knowing about these chemical concoctions is important because most couples have great difficulty transitioning from the passionate to the cuddled and committed.

THE BENEFITS OF SEX

Sexuality feeds and balances our life force. When experienced in a healthy, loving, giving manner, sex causes our minds and bodies to expand rather than contract.

Just in case Cynthia and I haven't inspired you enough yet to make a surge toward sex, weekly sex also:

- **Improves immunity because it can increase IgA by 30 percent.** IgA is an antibody I previously introduced you to and it's your first line of defense for colds and flu; it is the same antibody that increases with a positive mind-set (see page 132) and decreases with anger.[9]
- **Lowers blood pressure.** Sex twice a week reduces the risk of fatal heart attack by half.[10]
- **Burns 85 calories for each 30 minutes**–if you are so lucky![11]
- **Reduces pain and promotes sleep,** which I hope you realize by now are hugely energy positive.
- **Builds confidence and motivates you to eat better and exercise more;** ditto energy positive.
- **Brings relief to women suffering from migraines.**[12]
- **Decreases the occurrence of erectile dysfunction (ED).** According to the *American Journal of Medicine*, ED is twice as high in men who do not have sex once a week. For men having sex three or more times a week, erectile dysfunction was four times less likely to occur.[13]

FOR THE LADIES

Ladies, did you know that seminal fluid contains all the hormones and chemicals needed to fuel romance, lust, deep connection, and well-being?[14] That precious elixir, which gets absorbed by the vaginal wall, contains:

CYNTHIA'S CORNER

At least once a week in my practice, a female client comes in bemoaning the fact that she feels ashamed after having sex with an unavailable or commitment-avoidant person. It seems the sooner a woman has sex with someone, the greater the shame factor, especially if that person disappears soon after the sexual encounter. Even more disturbing is that other women, "friends," oftentimes step in and pick up the shame stick for a few extra licks.

When this happens I explore with the client how she has internalized society's beliefs concerning women and sex, and the term bad girl *gets intricately dissected. After some verbal purging by the client and some healthy feminist education from me, I usually have the client stand up and perform a few minutes of Throw It Away. We then work on creating a Screensaver of the client feeling strong, confident, and good about herself with a title that frees her of shame such as, "I can have the kind of sex I want and feel good about myself," or more simply put, "I Did It My Way."*

- **Testosterone** to pep you up
- **Dopamine** to fuel passion and delirium
- **Oxytocin** to promote milk production and uterine contractions and "kindle the cuddle"
- **Follicle-stimulating hormone and luteinizing hormone** to keep your menstrual cycles regular (both hormones are critical for fertility)
- **Beta endorphins** to calm the mind and body
- **Norepinephrine** to bring on excessive energy, exhilaration, and loss of appetite (good for managing body weight)

If you are in a safe, committed, intimate relationship, having consistent sexual intercourse enhances your sexual, hormonal health. But 45 percent of women have some form of sexual problems concerning low desire or difficulty achieving orgasm.[15] If you are struggling with these issues, here are a few things that can help:

- **Limit carbohydrates, cigarettes, and coffee** and eat more fish oils, dark chocolate (in moderation), nonstarchy fruits and vegetables, and lean protein.[16]

- **Take a multivitamin** that contains zinc, arginine, magnesium, and vitamins A, B, C, and E.
- **Perform exercises that promote bloodflow.**
- **Ask your physician** if any of the medications you might be taking can interfere with your sexual desire and performance, including some well-known antidepressants.

To provide the support your glands need to function optimally, eat plenty of the following foods:[17, 18, 19]

- **Warming and pungent foods and spices help increase circulation.** Try pepper, horseradish, cinnamon, fennel, ginger, garlic, onions, leeks, chives, and Indian spices such as turmeric, anise, and cardamom.
- **Soy products, pomegranate, and fennel** bind estrogen receptors and "help the vaginal area remain lubricated and combat symptoms of menopause–particularly hot flashes."[20] *Note:* Breast cancer survivors (including Cynthia) should use soy in moderation because it has been linked to breast cancer recurrence.
- **Asparagus,** which is high in vitamin E, may stimulate the production of testosterone.
- **Avocados** are high in folic acid, B_6, and potassium, which help build proteins, regulate thyroid function, and increase male hormone production.
- **Foods rich in L-arginine,** such as oatmeal, peanuts, walnuts, cashews, low-fat dairy, green and root veggies, soybeans, chickpeas, and seeds, are thought to increase desire in postmenopausal women.
- **Deep-sea, cold-water fish,** including salmon, halibut, sardines, mackerel, and shellfish, as well as fish oil capsules, contain nourishing omega-3 fatty acids.
- **Foods rich in essential fatty acids,** such as spinach, brown rice, wheat germ, pumpkin, nuts, olive oil, flax, and sesame seeds, provide lubrication for the skin, vagina, and eyes and are needed to produce female hormones.
- **Foods high in zinc,** such as oysters, liver, pork, beef, lamb, turkey, lentils, sesame seeds, pine nuts, and low-fat yogurt, help produce testosterone.
- **Eggs,** which are high in B_5 and B_6, are known to balance stress hormones.
- **Celery** contains the male hormone androsterone and has been shown to arouse women sexually.

- **Figs** contain many amino acids that may increase libido and sexual stamina.
- **Bananas** are high in bromelain, potassium, and B vitamins that help with testosterone production, and, well . . . look at the shape.

You'll see that the 7-Day Energy Surge eating plan already includes a lot of these foods, so not to worry, you'll get the fuel you need for your sexual energy soon enough!

In addition, of course, as we've already discussed, reaching your ideal weight will give you not only more energy but also more sexual confidence. As stated earlier in the book, as little as a 10 percent weight loss can boost your sex life. In fact, 30 percent of obese people seek help for sexual issues, and recent research shows that high cholesterol and insulin resistance can cause the arteries of the genitals to clog in both men and women, causing decreased bloodflow and less responsiveness. To make matters worse, the more body fat you have, the more SHBG (sex hormone binding globulin) you have, which binds to testosterone, making it less available to bring you lust and drive.[21]

That being said, however, you don't need to be "Beverly Hills Thin" to feel sexy and have a healthy sex life. In fact, society's highly distorted ideal body image in and of itself can reduce your libido. The average woman is not shaped like the 17-year-old, 6-foot-tall model, with inflated lips and a sliver of a nose, yet the desire to look like her is overwhelming for women of all ages. Not great for self-esteem, but very lucrative for plastic surgeons. Thank heaven for the current fabulous middle-aged female role models like Oprah, Diane Sawyer, Gloria Steinem, and J. K. Rowling, who demonstrate that grace, beauty, and self-acceptance are genuine possibilities. Self-acceptance of your body is a worthy goal at any weight, and by now you know what to do to promote more health and energy.

Dr. Susan Kellog, director of the Pelvic and Sexual Health Institute of Graduate Hospital in Philadelphia, says that women's decreasing sexual response with age stems from blockages in the tiny blood vessels leading to the clitoris that hamper bloodflow. As women age, the vaginal walls can thin and atrophy, which makes orgasms more difficult to achieve and less intense and can even cause intercourse to become painful.[22]

The following two exercises are based on Dr. Arnold Kegel's famous muscular contracting exercises to strengthen and control energy flow of the pubic floor, which is the area between the pubic bone and the tailbone. By regularly practicing these exercises, women

CYNTHIA'S CORNER

At 53, I am learning that moving my body is as important as eating right, and I sit all day for a living. With increased physical activity, I notice my skin is glowing, my hair is shining, my joints are more flexible, weight comes off easier, I have less bloat and, oh, well, other things I can't speak of as a working professional therapist. As my female clients exercise more, a task I usually assign as homework, they do report more interest in sex, increased arousal, and better self-confidence. Any of Jim's exercises, as well as yoga, brings increased bloodflow to the large muscles of the lower body that douse the genitals as well. I also recommend a Kegelesque exercise, modified by yours truly, that will strengthen the pelvic muscles near the vagina, bringing bloodflow specifically to the area. I call it the Costas/Karas Mula Bandha *(see page 170).*

can strengthen the vaginal muscles as well as those holding the vagina, uterus, and bladder. Kegels also:[23, 24]

- Bring bloodflow, lymphatic flow, and lubrication to the area for more pleasure and sensitivity
- Help achieve stronger orgasms
- Increase the thickness of the vaginal walls
- Increase bladder and bowel control
- Prevent or lessen the severity of urinary issues, such as stress incontinence
- Prevent or help vaginal and/or uterine prolapse[25]
- Speed healing from an episiotomy
- Reduce occurrence of hemorrhoids from childbirth
- Benefit pregnant women by preparing the area for childbirth stress and vaginal birth

COSTAS/KARAS MULA BANDHA

A mula bandha is a yogic term for a body position and/or muscle contraction that "has both energetic and physical effects," as well as "beneficial effects of breathing and the action of the nervous and endocrine systems," according to Guru Prem.[26] Whether you are currently having sex regularly or not, practice these exercises because they simulate orgasmic contractions and promote sexual vibrancy.

To locate the right set of muscles, there are three things you can do. First, sit on the toilet and partially empty your bladder, then try to stop the flow of urine and pay attention to the feeling of your deep muscles tensing. If at first you cannot stop the flow but can slow it down, don't worry. Do not do this often because it can cause problems with retaining urine, but every month or so you can check to see whether stopping the flow gets easier after practicing the techniques below. The second way to locate the muscles is to imagine that you are holding back gas. It should feel like a lifting up and a contraction without the use of your abdominal, leg, or buttock muscles. Thirdly, you can always insert a finger or two into your vagina and see whether you can squeeze your vaginal canal, or try it during sex with your partner. Breathe deeply and do not hold your breath. You will be doing two types of squeezes: one that holds the contraction for a certain amount of time and another type that is a series of quick contractions to strengthen the muscles that stop urination, especially when you sneeze or laugh.

Now, we're ready:

1. Put on some great stimulating music with a strong beat. Sit up in your bed with your back straight against the headboard and your legs straight out in front of you, feet about 12 inches apart.

2. Place one hand above your belly button and the other below.

3. Pull your chin back and slightly down so that your head rests between your shoulders and is not jutting forward.

4. Take two deep cleansing breaths that cause your hands to move up and outward.

5. Now, without moving your hands, squeeze your vaginal muscles upward and inward without tensing your buttocks and leg muscles.

6. Hold for a count of 5 and rest for a count of 5. Work up to a set of 25 contractions twice a day. When that gets easy, hold the contraction for a count of 10.

7. Alternate by doing 25 quick contractions, pause for 30 seconds, then work your way up to 100 quick pumps. Do this twice a day, too.

BUTTERFLY YOGA POSE

Another yoga position that can help activate and energize your passion playground is the butterfly.

1. Sit on the floor with your back straight and the outside of your thighs resting on the floor as you bring the soles of your feet together.

2. With your hands clasped together, cradle the soles of your feet, helping to hold your feet together and sit up straight. Bring your feet as close to your crotch as is comfortable and do not overstretch.

3. Take two cleansing breaths and gently bounce your knees up and down for 2 to 3 minutes. At first your thighs might not be able to touch the ground, but with practice your hip joints will loosen and your inner thighs will stretch and lengthen.

4. If possible, try to do this 15 minutes before sex.

There is a misconception that with menopause comes a halt of sexual desire and function. Although menopause may contribute to vaginal dryness and thinning, diminished libido *and* clitoral sensitivity, there does exist data that suggest women who remain sexually active suffer less from these symptoms. I guess it's the "use it or lose it" philosophy espoused by Masters and Johnson. Even the National Institute on Aging and the North American Menopause Society recommend that women keep having intercourse or masturbating regularly to "increase sexual responsiveness and pleasure."[27, 28] Guys, well, I think we have this covered.

And ladies, if you are a cougar, I applaud you!

FOR THE GUYS

Guys' issues with sex are a whole other story. First of all, most men *love* the chase and the conquest and then, frequently, soon thereafter, are, ah, done–fact of life, because that is somewhat the way we are wired. Then, for some, performance anxiety pops up (or is it pops down?), and trust me, it happens. If you keep reading, you will learn which foods can make a difference in your tumescence (one of my favorite words–it means "swelling" or "showing signs of swelling"). You will also learn how to become a good listener, which will get you more . . .

CYNTHIA'S CORNER

Dear Men: *Women's sexual desire is strongly linked to how they feel about their bodies and whether their mates help make them feel desirable and cherished. Many of my female clients complain that their mates wake up grumpy, criticize, and bark orders, and then 14 hours later expect these women to be lusting for them. What happens instead is that after spending most of the day replaying the negativity in their minds that caught them off guard first thing in the morning, resentment brews, tension mounts, and rebuttals are rehearsed, and the last thing these women want to do is open themselves up emotionally and physically to sex. I'm sure this happens with men, too, but it's a common complaint coming from women. Jim will provide some spicy information below, so don't stop reading now.*

Some men lack the verbal tools needed to establish intimacy and connection and usually learn the hard way, by frustrating and confusing the hell out of our partners. We don't know how to verbally express ourselves and often don't communicate what we are seeking—whether it be a one-night stand or a true interest in getting to know the other person. So guys, rule number one—be honest about your intentions, because hurting another person also comes with the consequences of karma, or "what goes around comes around." It's also an energy saboteur.

Here's a recommendation—pitch in. Dr. Joshua Coleman, author of *The Lazy Husband*, recommends joining your mate to clean and shop, because it will show your support as well as free up more time. More time equals more time for some action. Also, make sure you memorize the tips on date night etiquette that are coming up on page 176.

Now guys, we have some options to enhance *our* personal energy surge as well as our tumescence (there's that word again). Strong, healthy bloodflow is our greatest friend (yes!) in the bedroom (besides our mates). Eating the right foods, which happen to be the same foods that prevent heart disease and diabetes, is a must. So consume more:[29]

- **Pomegranate juice.** A study in the *Journal of Urology* found that it removed the risk of erectile dysfunction in rabbits. You know how I feel about juice, so I'm talking one glass of sparkling ice water with 1 or 2 ounces of juice!

- **Blueberries.** Good fiber and plenty of antioxidants help rid the body of toxins and move out cholesterol from the digestive tract.
- **Spinach.** Japanese researchers found that the large amount of magnesium in spinach keeps blood vessels dilated, and you know what that's good for. Remember, magnesium also helps the body preserve lean muscle tissue, and we all know what Popeye looks like.
- **Citrus fruit.** Higher sperm counts are found in men who consume 2,000 milligrams of vitamin C a day. In addition, vitamin C prevents sperm from clumping, so they can "swim solo" more efficiently upstream and get their job done.
- **Oatmeal.** Oats have a chemical that releases testosterone in the bloodstream, thus invigorating orgasm and fueling sex drive. Girls, I think you should eat this, too!
- **Shrimp salad.** Shrimp contains a lot of zinc, and leafy vegetables contain folate; together they act to increase sperm count for those looking to conceive. FYI, folate helps reduce inflammation.
- **Honey.** B vitamins in honey assist in the production of testosterone; honey's boron content assists estrogen in promoting arousal and bloodflow. Consider using it sparingly to sweeten your antioxidant-rich coffee or tea.

Note: Men, we can also benefit from doing Kegels, which have been known to help with prostatic pain, swelling, and urinary incontinence, as well as help achieve stronger erections.

FOR COUPLES

What if you are always tired, drained, exhausted, and depleted to the point where you avoid sexual intimacy? We all have a say and a power when it comes to our sex lives, and I

Body Weight and Fertility

According to a study presented at the annual conference of the European Society of Human Reproduction and Embryology, men considered obese (which means a BMI of 30 or more) are 40 percent more likely to have sperm abnormalities and 60 percent more likely to have less semen, both reducing the chances of a successful egg fertilization. The researchers theorize that excess fat raises the testicles' temperature and may interfere with sperm production and quality.[30]

CYNTHIA'S CORNER

During the course of my professional career, I've noticed that the quality of lust, longing, and sexual desire described at the start of this chapter rarely lasts more than a few years for most couples. With the passing of time comes familiarity and routine, stress, past sexual trauma, children, finances, medical issues, work, and everyday life; couples are all too aware of their decreased libido and less frequent good times in the bedroom. This unfortunate situation brings with it emotions of insecurity, anger, resentment, embarrassment, and the fear that perhaps you are no longer in love or that your mate is no longer in love with you. What couples need to know is that the bonding hormones are very strong, and if couples can create a safe haven where they can come together to discuss their hurts and sorrows, their goals and dreams, side by side, life can be both comfortable and exciting. We provide you with many different pathways for a smoother road toward love and togetherness.

bet there was a time in your life when you had a more satisfying, active, adventurous sex life. I also would bet that you possessed more *energy* at that same time.

According to Peggy Vaughan's book, *The Monogamy Myth*, 60 percent of males and 40 percent of females will have an affair over the course of a relationship. You'd better nip this potential problem in the bud and work on your sexual energy's wavelength, vibration, and pulsation. Here are some simple things you can do to keep the spark alive.

Touch Each Other

Someone very wise once said, "Sex starts in the morning," and guys, I am not referring to our morning male physiology here. What I am speaking about are the first words, actions, and behavior toward your partner when you open your eyes in the morning. These initial communications will determine the tone of your relationship throughout the day and, most important, later that evening. Mornings are a crucial time to mutually kindle each other's energy.

Upon waking, give a tender hug or caress, a few moments of rubbing your partner's back, or words of love and appreciation that will leave your mate feeling nurtured, desired, and wanting to reconnect that evening.

Young lab rats that were gently and consistently touched grew more and were faster learners than those that were not handled. Rats that were also deprived of food and touch opted for touch when given a choice. We all know that orphaned children who lacked physical affection in infancy have lower intelligence and stunted physical growth. When you touch your partner, you are raising his or her levels of chemicals responsible for growth, relaxation, and respiration, thereby promoting health, longevity, and energy. On a quick note, the relaxation response is also triggered by seeing your partner smile and/or hearing his/her soft or soothing voice, compliments of the vagal nerve.[31] Won't bore you with the physiology.

Kiss

Another common complaint that Cynthia and I hear from both sexes is, "We just don't kiss like we used to." Did you know that your lips are one of the areas of your body most densely populated with sensory neurons and that a very large portion of your brain's cortex is devoted to your lips? They must be pretty important!

In a recent study presented at the Society of Neuroscience, kissing was shown to reduce stress because it lowered cortisol levels in both sexes, and by now you know cortisol is an energy killer. Kissing was also found to deepen breathing, dilate pupils, and subdue rational thought and self-consciousness–plus, plus, plus.[32]

Researchers at Lafayette College found that kissing releases that cuddle hormone oxytocin (which I previously described) and decreases cortisol.[33] In a study published in the *Journal of Sexuality Research and Social Policy*, couples that had frequent kissing sessions were more satisfied and committed in their relationships.[34]

If you aren't convinced by now, how about the fact that for every 10 minutes of kissing you burn 11 calories (and can't possibly get anything else in your mouth to eat or drink), so start kissing again and throw caution to the wind.[35]

Play Together

It is found that couples who do some type of physical activity together have better sex lives, too. Cynthia and I have discussed that the couples we know who play golf or tennis, dance, ski, or work out together all seem to be having more sex. If you really want to build and promote feelings of romance and attraction, scientists have found that doing "novel" activities together (Did I hear tango lessons?) actually elevates your dopamine levels even higher and boosts brain neuroplasticity.[36]

Ever notice the embrace and rapture of couples who have just bungee-jumped together? The activity doesn't have to be that fear producing, but taking vacations to exciting places, surprising each other with theater tickets, or trying new restaurants are all ways of creating novelty–the unexpected.

Although you want to spend quality time together, you also want to give each other the space to breathe (you know how important breathing is, right?). When your partner is in need of solitude, or you are presently single, then work on yourself–relaxing, reaching out to friends, trying a healthy new recipe, practicing yoga, meditating, creating a new music mix, or taking a class–try anything new and exciting, but *not* a group exercise class!

Have Date Nights

We've all heard about the necessity of scheduling a weekly "date night," especially those of us with kids. It's a great concept, but there need to be some date night guidelines, or your squabbles and differences will follow you out the door. Cynthia and I came up with the etiquette of date night:

- Listen to each other and take the time to acknowledge what your mate is saying. Do not give advice.
- No talking about the kids, in-laws, or money!
- If double-dating, go out with happy couples who have a healthy relationship (i.e., leave Heather Mills and Paul McCartney at home).
- Every so often, bring along two pads of paper and write down 25 things you want to do, have, or become. Then combine what you like from each other's lists to create a "couple's list." *Note:* Be supportive of your mate's list!

Natural Pheromones

Back in Elizabethan times, couples flaunted their pheromones, in contrast to our society's use of perfumes, deodorizers, douches, sachets, you name it—anything to mask our natural body odors. Back in the day, a woman used to place a peeled apple in her armpit to absorb her scent, then send it to her lover to sniff in her absence. I know that sounds "out there," but it's true. Can you even imagine the look on your partner's face when such a gift arrives?

- **Don't overeat.** How sexy do you feel with a hunk of pasta, meat, fries, or pizza swelling your gut upward and outward? Even better idea: Have sex before dinner. Don't underestimate the power of the "quickie."
- **Talk to your mate** about the good old times as you listen to music (remember all the positives from the previous component). Another recent study showed that reminiscing about good times helped couples make up easier after a fight, so perhaps you can listen to music and reminisce for a double whammy.
- **Take it easy on the deodorant and the perfume,** because they can mask our precious pheromones. Bathing is better, and bathing "togetha is mo' betta."

Bathe Together

During rough and rocky times, the benefits of water therapy, such as a bath, Jacuzzi, or hot shower, cannot be emphasized enough. Recall the benefits of cold water for relieving depression. Ever wonder why you feel so great during and after a visit to the beach or a dip in the pool? In one study published in the *Journal of Personality and Social Psychology*, 55 percent of the participants reported successful results from water therapy in lowering their stress levels and increasing their energy.[37] Water strikes again for energy!

When bathing, treat yourself to luxuriously rich and fragrant body washes, scrubs, and/or oils. Massage your partner's body and practice on each other what feels good in terms of pressure and speed of stroke. Afterward, visualize any toxins and negativity moving down the drain and away from your bodies.

Communicate

If you and your mate have difficulty communicating or cannot resolve a conflict, use this tried-and-true communication tool taught by Harville Hendrix, a master of couples therapy whom Cynthia studied under.

First decide who will be the speaker and who will be the listener. The person that is usually more quiet should be the first one to speak.

1. Sit facing your mate and ask him to tell you in detail something that's bothering him. Once the speaker starts, the listener is quiet.

CYNTHIA'S CORNER

I'd be lost without this technique in couple's therapy. When couples first come in, they are so angry and frustrated from years of unsuccessful communication that invariably during the first session, one member stands up, throws up his/her hands, hurls expletives, and threatens to leave. Immediately, I put my Hendrix hat on, silence them, seat them facing each other, and teach them this beloved technique. It's almost magical to witness both parties melt throughout the process, begin to feel more connected and understood, and later walk out the door holding hands.

2. The speaker must use "I" statements and not blame the other partner or use the word *you* in any way. Tone of voice must be kind and gentle.

3. After a few minutes of the speaker talking, the listener says, "Let me see if I have this right . . ." and tries to repeat verbatim what she just heard.

4. The listener then asks the speaker, "Did I get that right?"

5. Now the speaker can add or correct what he needs in order to be understood. This can go on for a while until the speaker feels heard (though the listener may not necessarily agree).

6. The listener tells the speaker one thing she appreciates about him, and then the partners switch roles.

Although it appears easy, this exercise can be daunting, because both parties must maintain self-control. The speaker may not accuse and point fingers, and the listener may not comment on or analyze what has been said to him/her.

To further motivate you to practice expressing your emotions in a healthy way, researchers at the University of Michigan School of Public Health found that couples who express their feelings live longer than those who bury their emotions. The study also found that bottling up emotions led to anger, resentment, and a twofold increase in death from all causes.[38, 39]

Jealousy, insecurity, and clinginess are critical problems that impede the loving energy flow for both sexes. Mates can get overpowering and demanding, too, so I always refer to the following words of Rainer Maria Rilke, who I think would have been a terrific couples' therapist:

> "Once the realization is accepted that even between the closest of human beings infinite distances continue, a wonderful living side by side can grow up, if they succeed in loving the distance between them which makes it possible for each to see the other whole against the sky." And in a separate quote he said, "A good marriage is that in which each appoints the other guardian of his solitude."

I interpret this as, "I want for us to be two wholes that come together and are interesting, multifaceted, and complementary, as we agree and accept that we are going to journey together and sometimes alone."

> *Note:* For both singles and couples–don't nurture with your old friends Ben on one side of the bed and Jerry on the other, who feel good going down but not so good the next morning when you step on the scale. Try water therapy instead.

FOR THE SINGLETON

Lately I've noticed how many of my married friends and coworkers long to be single. If you are single and happy in your life, kudos to you. If you are single and wanting to be in a relationship, enjoy your time without constraints until you meet the right one. Work on filling yourself up from the inside out and realize that there *are* ways you can work on your sexuality yourself. Here are a few of those ways.

Be Kind to Yourself

Monitor how you define and label yourself, and scan for negativity and self-deprecation. What do you say to yourself first thing in the morning? Are you kind and warm to yourself and filled with enthusiasm for the coming day, or do you wake up and immediately self-attack with some "mustabatory" statements, such as "I must get married"? Remember, a good day doesn't happen by chance–you MAKE it happen. Get up and give yourself a 2-minute scalp massage. Take a minute to place your two index fingers on the bones behind your ears and press and rub in a circular motion, then grab an ear in each hand and knead away.

Try pulling your knees up to your chest, hug them with both hands, and roll side-to-side to stretch out your back. Remember, one huge benefit of being single is that you get the whole bed to stretch out in.

Touch Yourself

Learning how to touch and show affection to yourself and others takes practice and patience. If your parents rarely touched you or each other, it might be uncomfortable and/or foreign to you. The skin (which happens to be the largest organ of the body) is the first layer of our nervous system and if gently stroked can enhance and stimulate us in wonderful ways. Remember what that cold shower can do for your mood?

Once again, for you singles, any kind of therapeutic touch promotes well-being. If you can't go to a spa or health club or have a massage therapist come to your home, there are many massage schools that offer discounted massage by students in training, and they are frequently very good. If you are an adventurer, try acupressure or Feldenkrais. I mentioned the pluses of acupuncture and Feldenkrais in Component 8, De-Stress to Surge.

And remember that bathing is a great time to practice gentle touches. When bathing, treat yourself to luxuriously rich and fragrant body washes, scrubs, and/or oils. Massage your body and practice on yourself what feels good in terms of pressure and speed of stroke. Afterward, visualize any toxins and negativity moving away from your body and down the drain.

Try New Things

If you are single, there are many ways of creating novelty in your life; go on an outing to a museum, take a dance class, join a book club or network for single people, or take a foreign language class. Push yourself to try something new every week. It will keep you moving, increase testosterone and dopamine levels in your blood, create new brain cells, bring you "out there," and, most important, keep you young. Remember, dopamine boosts creativity, spontaneity, curiosity, and *energy*. Become an adventurer and an explorer. It's so much easier being single these days, because marriage is getting such a bad rap with the highest divorce rate ever.

Learn to Listen

If you are single, you can still use the active listening approach mentioned on pages 177–178. Practice this with your close friends, because it really teaches you how to listen. According to contemporary author and spiritual teacher Ram Dass, "The quieter you become, the more you will hear." This will get you into the habit of expressing what you need and desire clearly, which will not only help if and when you do find a mate, but will also help your relationships with your family, friends, colleagues, and anyone else.

To sum up, sex can be a wonderfully therapeutic, healthy, energizing pursuit if you have a loving partner or are truly interested in "romantic" dating. If you are newly involved, please try to enjoy the early stages of "crazy love," and just know that you will be somewhat psycho for the first 6 to 18 months due to your chemicals of lust and attraction. It's the ultimate roller-coaster ride, and if you hang in there long enough, the roller coaster will probably become a cruise–a cruise with both smooth *and* rocky waters. Enjoy the bonding stage and create a beautiful, safe, secure nest together to house your love.

If you are married or in a long-term, committed relationship, schedule your date nights and follow the dating rules of etiquette. Make sure you schedule your sexual encounters as well, so they don't get lost in the vagaries of life. Staying connected is crucial to any relationship's *energy* state.

If you are currently single and searching for love, read about it, talk about it, and stay open and positive to possibilities; you are in charge of your life. Set your course to new and exciting destinations, and bask in your current freedom to go and do as you please.

To all, take care of your mind and body through healthy movement and nutritious foods, and try to make that extra effort to look your best for yourself as well as others. Massage your skin with fragrant lotions, use water and music to soothe yourself, tell yourself you are beautiful, and then tell someone else. You know the expression "You get what you give"? Live by it.

PART II

THE 7-DAY ENERGY SURGE PLAN

PREPARATION

Now that you've learned all about the 10 components of energy and how they work together to fire up your senses, boost your metabolism, and get your brain humming, it's time to put them to work for you. I suggest that you start the 7-Day Energy Surge plan on a Monday, so that you can use the weekend before to prepare. Once you begin the plan, you'll see that there are a number of things you'll be doing every day (including breathing, working on your mind-set, and performing de-stressing exercises) and some that you'll do on only a few days (including exercising). I've specified which days to do those, but if you find that you need to move those pieces around due to your schedule, you can certainly do just that.

Now let's get started!

❒ Take the Energy Surge Quiz on page xvi.

RECORD YOUR OVERALL SCORE HERE:

❒ Write down the two categories in which you scored the highest: ________ ________

❒ Write down the two categories in which you scored the lowest: ________ ________

READ, OBSERVE, AND RECORD THE FOLLOWING:

❒ Read through the 7-Day Energy Surge plan and decide when you want to do each exercise.

❒ Complete the following sentence:

When I was lighter, ____

❒ Count your breath cycles per minute and determine your balance of shallow to deep breathing. Record your results here: ______________

❒ Create and title your Screensaver. My Screensaver is named: ______________

❒ Schedule both sleep and wake-up times for the next 7 days.

	Bedtime	Wake-Up Time
Monday		
Tuesday		
Wednesday		
Thursday		
Friday		

	Bedtime	Wake-Up Time
Saturday		
Sunday		

❒ If you have been keeping one, review your food diary. If not, start one now. Just recording what you eat during this weekend will help you determine where you have difficulty with your eating habits. Plan a strategy to address these issues.

❒ Observe how you behave toward yourself first thing in the morning. Do you think about all the things you're looking forward to in your day, or do you start worrying about what you should have done yesterday?

❒ If you are married or in a committed relationship, observe how you behave toward your mate first thing in the morning. Are you kind and loving, or do you bound out of bed and either start to bark orders ("Where are my keys?") or ignore each other and run off to get a jump-start on your day?

SET YOUR SLEEP STAGE:

❒ Assess your mattress—If it is more than 5 or 10 years old or you are having back pain first thing in the morning, you definitely need a new one.

❒ Assess your pillows—If they are more than a year old or if you are waking up with neck pain, you need new ones.

❒ Assess your sheets, which should be soft and keep you cool.

❒ If you don't already have them, buy earplugs, a sleep mask, snore strips (if your mate snores), and a dim night-light for your bathroom.

❒ Buy your pet(s) their own beds, and start to train them to use them. This will most likely take longer than 7 days, but at least you will get a jump-start.

MAKE SURE YOU HAVE EVERYTHING YOU NEED FOR THE SURGE:

❒ Find a space in your home with a door and enough space around it where you can perform the full exercise program. I recommend that you have a clock with a large second hand in view in this room.

❐ Buy a braided SPRI StrengthCord and door attachment (where to buy them is listed on page 69).

❐ If you have a scale, take it out and put it in your bathroom or bedroom and make sure it is in working order. If it isn't or you don't own one, buy one.

❐ If you ever played an instrument that you blow into, find it, take it out, and clean it. If not, go buy a harmonica.

❐ Make sure your stereo and iPod are in working order. If they're not, get them fixed.

❐ Make a playlist of energetic music you'd like to listen to in the morning and another playlist of soothing music you'd like to listen to as you fall asleep.

❐ Take out the smallest plates and cups you own.

❐ Purge all junk food and drinks from your kitchen.

❐ Investigate whether there is a place to buy wheatgrass juice near your home or office. If not, buy Green Magma, Greens+, Kyo-Green, or freeze-dried wheatgrass that you add to water.

❐ Make sure you bring sparkling water to your workplace so that you have plenty on hand to drink whenever you want.

❐ Make the Bieler's Broth (page 189).

❐ Now, go grocery shopping.

SHOPPING LIST

As I discussed earlier, I'd really like you to try to follow the eating plan as much as possible, but I understand that it can be difficult when you're really busy. In general, I don't want you wasting your precious energy shopping and cooking, because you have much more important things to do this week, so I made this plan simple. You only need 38 ingredients, and the meals are easy to make. You may be able to just grocery shop once, on the Saturday or Sunday before your Monday start, or you may think it best to shop again around Thursday if you feel that you are sacrificing freshness for convenience. If, after reading through the plan, you feel that it's still too much for you to do, you can just find one or two meals you like and think you can stick with, and simply repeat those. See the substitutions on page 189 for more ideas on how you can simplify the plan to work for you.

Note: You will have some leftover, nonperishable ingredients for the following week.

Dairy

Eggs = 2 dozen
Feta = 4 ounces
Sargento low-fat Cheddar slices = 1 small package
Low-fat yogurt = 4 containers, 100 calories each
String cheese, low fat = 3 pieces
1% or 2% cottage cheese = one 8-ounce container

Packaged foods

Whole wheat or whole grain bread = 1 loaf (just make sure the bread is 80 calories or less per slice)
Lärabar = 2
Almonds = 60 unsalted
Oatmeal = three 40-gram packs, either instant or old-fashioned
Kraft Light Done Right Red Wine Vinaigrette = 1 small bottle
Peanut butter = 1 small jar (natural or organic would be best but is not required)
Dijon mustard = 1 small jar
Balsamic vinegar = 1 small bottle
Corn tortillas = 1 small package; you will need a total of 4
Pickles = 1 small jar

Produce

Red bell pepper = about 3, or enough for 5 cups
Tomato = about 3, or enough for 5¼ cups
Red onion = 1 large, or enough for 2¼ cups
Spinach = two 10-ounce bags, or enough for 3 cups
Zucchini = 2 whole
Blueberries = 16 ounces, or enough for 2 cups
Mixed greens = five 10-ounce bags, or enough for 16 salads
Bananas = 2
Broccoli = 3 heads, or enough for 5 cups
Cucumbers = 2, or enough for 3 cups
Apples = 3 whole
Celery = 3 stalks
Lemons or limes = 6

Ingredients for Bieler's Broth

Parsley = 3 bunches
Green beans = 1½ pounds
Zucchini = 2½ pounds

Meat

Low-fat sliced turkey breast = ½ pound, or enough for 11 thin slices
Chicken breast = 21 ounces
Shrimp = 8 ounces
Salmon = 10 ounces
Tuna steak = 8 ounces
Steak (for steak salad) = 4 ounces

Nonperishables

Cooking spray
Salt
Pepper
Ketchup
Mustard
Lemon juice
Chili powder
Garlic powder
A case of sparkling water

BIELER'S BROTH

A Potent, Energy-Expanding Elixir

3 bunches of parsley, rinsed very well and stems cut off

1½ pounds green beans, ends cut off

2½ pounds zucchini, ends cut off and sliced into chunks

Place the parsley, green beans, and zucchini in a big pot, then add enough water to just cover the vegetables. Bring to a boil, cover, and simmer for 30 minutes, until a fork easily pierces the zucchini. Let cool, then puree in batches in a blender or food processor, adding in some of the vitamin-rich water. The consistency should resemble pea soup.

This recipe should make approximately 21 cups, or enough for all 7 days of the Surge. Ideally, keep it in a glass container, cutting back on the plastic, which it is not good for your health or the environment.

Note: Do not add any salt, seasoning, or anything else to this sacred, medicinal potion.

Substitutions

1. Meals. If you simply don't have the time to prepare some of the items on the menu, here are simple substitution meals.

Breakfast

1 packet of instant oatmeal or ½ cup cottage cheese and one piece of fruit

or

¾ cup of non-sugar-added cereal and ½ cup 1% milk

Lunch

Turkey sandwich on whole wheat bread with lettuce, tomato, and Dijon mustard

or

4 cups of vegetables topped with 6 ounces of grilled chicken, shrimp, or fish and plain balsamic vinegar

Dinner

6 ounces of lean protein: boneless, skinless chicken or turkey, lean meat, fish, or seafood

3 cups of steamed vegetables

One medium-size baked or sweet potato with salt and pepper

or

3 cups of greens

1 hard-boiled egg

4 ounces of lean turkey or chicken

2 ounces of Swiss or Cheddar cheese

Balsamic vinegar

Note: As I mentioned in Component 2, this eating plan gives 1,200 calories a day. Men need to add 200 additional calories a day. This can be accomplished by adding the appropriate portion of the following:

- One serving of fruit, which is 100 calories and defined as one medium-size piece or ½ cup cut up
- An additional egg—90 calories
- An additional yogurt—generally 100 calories
- 4 additional ounces of grilled chicken—approximately 180 calories
- A few more of the approved ingredients in the 7-Day Eating Surge in a portion-controlled manner

2. **Dairy.** For those of you who are lactose intolerant, I recommend that you replace many of the dairy products in this plan with hard cheeses, such as Swiss and Cheddar, which possess far less lactose. Use soy, rice, almond, or lactose-free milk, or add a lactase supplement to meals or the actual milk product to reduce symptoms.
3 **Nuts.** If you are allergic to nuts, then eliminate all nuts and peanut butter and replace the exact calorie count with another source of protein. For example, a rolled-up deli turkey slice with a little Dijon mustard is a tasty, filling substitution, and it is already part of the eating plan. I also recommend snacking on legumes, such as chickpeas. As I said, I do that with my kids all the time.
4. **Vegetarian.** If you're vegetarian, then replace the animal protein with low-fat dairy, legumes, or tofu. Just be vigilant in keeping the calorie count exactly the same.
5. **Eggs.** There are some people who avoid eggs due to their reputation for high cholesterol, which is approximately 210 milligrams per yolk. But, a study conducted at Harvard University in 1999 did not find a link between one egg a day and heart disease, with the exception of those with diabetes.[17] Therefore, you shouldn't fear eggs, because there is also some evidence that eggs promote a feeling of fullness as a result of the protein and fat content, and I already said that I think they are the ideal

A Word from Our Testers

"I feel terrific! It really took until yesterday to start feeling things kick into gear, and today I have a ton of energy!"

—*Colleen M., age 39*

postworkout snack. If you are still not convinced that eggs are right for you, then substitute two egg whites for every whole egg, or try a product such as Egg Beaters With Yolk, which contains less fat and cholesterol than the real thing but tastes great.

6. **Eating out.** If possible, try the 7-Day Energy Surge during a week when you can cook for yourself, so that you can follow the menus here exactly and get used to eating simply and in smaller portions. If you absolutely have to eat out, though, please have a plan. I love the phrase "A failure to plan is a plan to fail." If you are eating out, then you must check out the Web site for the restaurant you are going to and see whether they list the calories (and sodium content) of their meals.

A Word from Our Testers

"I would recommend cooking all the chicken and meats and chopping all the vegetables ahead of time to save time during the busy week."

—Colleen M., age 39

"The first few days may be tough, but hang in there. And do allow enough time in the beginning and end of the day, even 15 minutes, to do all of the exercises."

—Andrew M., age 41

Note: All national chain restaurants in New York are now required to do so by law (thanks, Mayor Bloomberg) right on the menu. You will be shocked and horrified when you see the calorie count of many of your favorites, including choices you thought were lower in calories. Just a visit to a New York Starbucks alone will astound you.

If the restaurant is not a chain and their menu is not on the Web, then call and ask them to fax a menu in advance. Search for words such as *poached*, *steamed*, *broiled*, and *baked*, and have a game plan going in. Poached salmon and steamed vegetables will keep you right on target. Just don't go in without a strategy in place and, at the very least, nix the breadbasket.

Note: I give you even more recommendations on dining out on page 224.

If you do elect to make these changes, then adjust the shopping list accordingly.

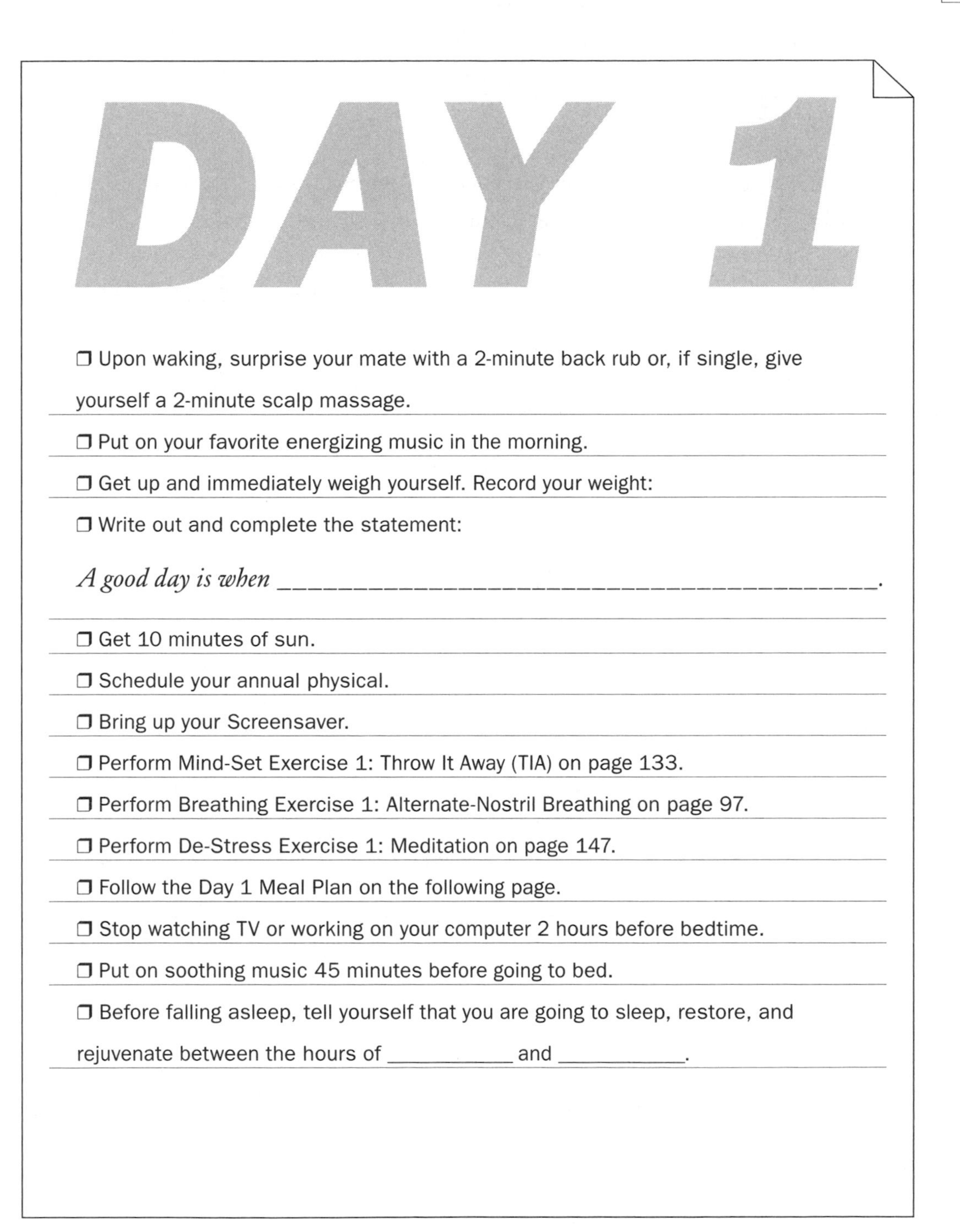

DAY 1

❐ Upon waking, surprise your mate with a 2-minute back rub or, if single, give yourself a 2-minute scalp massage.

❐ Put on your favorite energizing music in the morning.

❐ Get up and immediately weigh yourself. Record your weight:

❐ Write out and complete the statement:

A good day is when ______________________________________.

❐ Get 10 minutes of sun.

❐ Schedule your annual physical.

❐ Bring up your Screensaver.

❐ Perform Mind-Set Exercise 1: Throw It Away (TIA) on page 133.

❐ Perform Breathing Exercise 1: Alternate-Nostril Breathing on page 97.

❐ Perform De-Stress Exercise 1: Meditation on page 147.

❐ Follow the Day 1 Meal Plan on the following page.

❐ Stop watching TV or working on your computer 2 hours before bedtime.

❐ Put on soothing music 45 minutes before going to bed.

❐ Before falling asleep, tell yourself that you are going to sleep, restore, and rejuvenate between the hours of ___________ and ___________.

DAY 1

DAY 1 MEAL PLAN
1,204 CALORIES

In addition to the meals below, consume 3 cups of Bieler's Broth, 3+ cups of tea, and no more than 300 milligrams of caffeine in either tea or coffee after noon.

Breakfast — Greek Omelet = 289 calories

5 egg whites = 75

1 ounce feta cheese = 74

1 cup chopped spinach = 8

1 cup chopped red pepper = 26

½ cup chopped tomato = 19

Salt and pepper

Cooking spray = 7

1 slice whole wheat toast = 80

Combine the egg whites, feta, spinach, red pepper, chopped tomato, and salt and pepper to taste. Coat the inside of a nonstick skillet with cooking spray and turn the heat to medium-high. Add the mixture. When the bottom side of the omelet is solid, flip or fold it over with a spatula and cook until the other side is done. Eat it with the toast.

Snack — Low-fat yogurt = 100 calories

Lunch — Grilled Turkey, Tomato, and Cheese Sandwich = 301 calories

Cooking spray = 7

2 slices whole wheat toast = 160

4 slices low-fat turkey = 46

2 slices tomato = 16

1 slice Sargento reduced-fat medium Cheddar = 60

3 pickle spears = 12

Coat the inside of a nonstick skillet with cooking spray. Grill one side of each slice of whole wheat bread until light brown. Add the turkey, tomato, and cheese. Serve with the pickle spears alongside.

Snack — Hard-boiled egg = 90 calories

Dinner — Chicken Skewers = 340 calories

4 ounces boneless, skinless chicken breast = 192

1 cup seeded and sliced red pepper = 26

1 cup sliced red onion = 60

1 large zucchini, sliced = 62

Salt and pepper

Prepare a grill or preheat the oven to 400°F. Cut the chicken, pepper, red onion, and zucchini into 1-inch pieces. Place on skewers, alternating all ingredients. Season with salt and pepper to taste and grill until chicken is cooked through.

Snack — 12 almonds = 84 calories

DAY 2

❒ Put on your favorite energizing music in the morning.

❒ Get up and immediately weigh yourself. Record your weight:

❒ Write and finish the statement:

A good day is when ______________________________.

❒ Get 10 minutes of sun.

❒ Schedule a date with your mate, or if single, book a massage.

❒ Bring up your Screensaver.

❒ Call a friend and "go public," as we talked about on page 7.

❒ Perform Mind-Set Exercise 2: Pat Yourself on the Back on page 134.

❒ Perform Breathing Exercise 2: Breathing into Blackness on page 98.

❒ Perform De-Stress Exercise 2: Tapping to Happy on page 148.

❒ Follow the 7-Day Exercise Program on pages 72–87. This exercise program should be performed 3 days a week on nonconsecutive days. During this 7-day plan, I've scheduled your exercise on Days 2, 4, and 6. If you need to change that to fit your schedule, that's fine, but keep in mind that the program is a full body workout, and therefore requires 48 hours of rest before you perform the routine again.

❒ Follow the Day 2 Meal Plan on the following page.

❒ Stop watching TV or working on your computer 2 hours before bedtime.

❒ Put on soothing music 45 minutes before going to bed.

❒ Before falling asleep, tell yourself that you are going to sleep, restore, and rejuvenate between the hours of ___________ and ___________.

DAY
2

DAY 2 MEAL PLAN
1,217 CALORIES

In addition to the meals below, consume 3 cups of Bieler's Broth, 3+ cups of tea, and no more than 300 milligrams of caffeine in either tea or coffee by noon.

Breakfast — Fruit and yogurt = 164 calories

Low-fat yogurt = 100

2 cups blueberries = 64

Combine ingredients and serve.

Snack — 1 Lärabar = 220 calories

Lunch — Lettuce Wraps = 318 calories

4 ounces cooked boneless, skinless, chicken breast, sliced = 192

½ cup chopped red onion = 30

½ cup chopped tomato = 19

1 ounce feta cheese = 74

2 lettuce leaves = 3

Salt and pepper

Roll the cooked chicken, red onion, tomatoes, and feta in the lettuce leaves. Season with salt and pepper.

Snack — 1 pack oatmeal = 100 calories

Dinner — Grilled Steak Salad = 335 calories

4 ounces filet mignon = 232

3 cups mixed greens = 24

½ cup chopped tomato = 19

¼ cup chopped red onion = 15

2 tablespoons Kraft Light Done Right Red Wine Vinaigrette = 45

Heat the grill. Grill the steak; slice. Combine the greens, tomatoes, and onion in a bowl. Top with the grilled steak slices and drizzle with the red wine vinaigrette.

Snack 1 string cheese = 80 calories

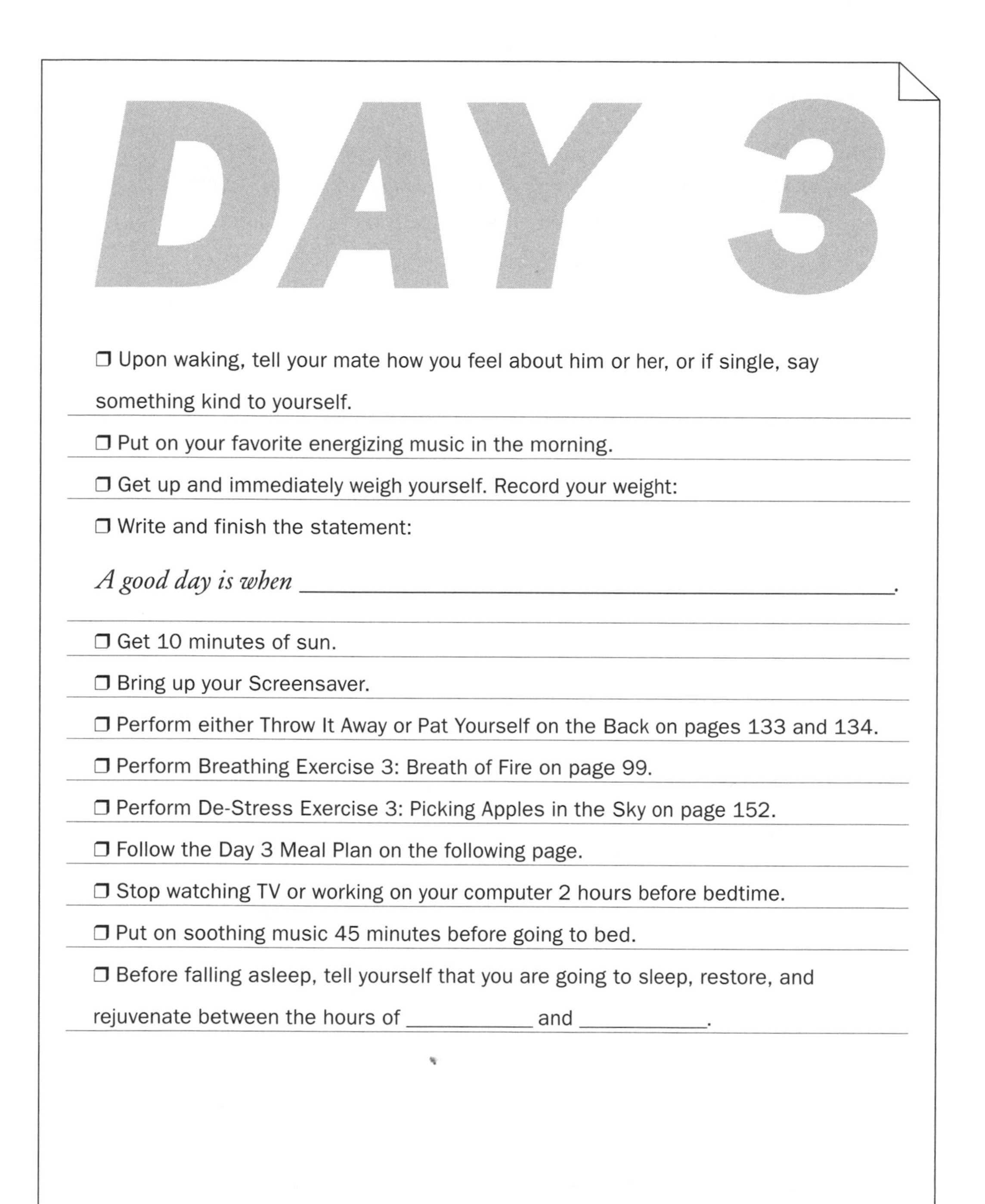

DAY 3

❒ Upon waking, tell your mate how you feel about him or her, or if single, say something kind to yourself.

❒ Put on your favorite energizing music in the morning.

❒ Get up and immediately weigh yourself. Record your weight:

❒ Write and finish the statement:

A good day is when ________________________________.

❒ Get 10 minutes of sun.

❒ Bring up your Screensaver.

❒ Perform either Throw It Away or Pat Yourself on the Back on pages 133 and 134.

❒ Perform Breathing Exercise 3: Breath of Fire on page 99.

❒ Perform De-Stress Exercise 3: Picking Apples in the Sky on page 152.

❒ Follow the Day 3 Meal Plan on the following page.

❒ Stop watching TV or working on your computer 2 hours before bedtime.

❒ Put on soothing music 45 minutes before going to bed.

❒ Before falling asleep, tell yourself that you are going to sleep, restore, and rejuvenate between the hours of ___________ and ___________.

DAY 3

DAY 3 MEAL PLAN
1,195 CALORIES

In addition to the meals below, consume 3 cups of Bieler's Broth, 3+ cups of tea, and no more than 300 milligrams of caffeine in either tea or coffee after noon.

Breakfast — Banana and Peanut Butter Oatmeal = 300 calories

1 packet plain instant oatmeal = 100

1 medium banana, sliced = 105

1 tablespoon peanut butter = 95

Mix the oatmeal, banana slices, and peanut butter, and microwave as directed on the package.

Snack — Low-fat yogurt = 100 calories

Lunch — Grilled Chicken Salad = 400 calories

3 cups mixed greens = 24

4 ounces cooked boneless, skinless chicken breast = 192

½ cup chopped tomato = 19

1 cup diced cucumber = 14

¼ cup chopped red onion = 15

1 cup chopped red pepper = 26

1 hard-boiled egg, sliced = 90

Salt and pepper

2 tablespoons balsamic vinegar = 20

Combine the greens, cooked chicken, tomato, cucumber, onion, red pepper, and hard-boiled egg in a bowl. Season with salt and pepper, and drizzle with balsamic vinegar.

Snack — 3 pieces rolled-up low-fat turkey with half sliced tomato and 1 tablespoon Dijon mustard = 97 calories

Dinner — Poached or Grilled Salmon = 311 calories

6 ounces skinless salmon fillet = 240

Salt and pepper

1 tablespoon lemon juice = 4

1 large zucchini = 67

Place the salmon in an 8" × 8" baking dish. Sprinkle with salt and pepper. Add water to the dish. Cover and cook in the microwave on high for 8 minutes, or until the fish turns opaque throughout and flakes easily when tested with a fork. Alternatively, grill the fish. Sprinkle with the lemon juice. Slice the zucchini and steam it to desired doneness. Serve with the fish.

Snack — 12 almonds = 84 calories

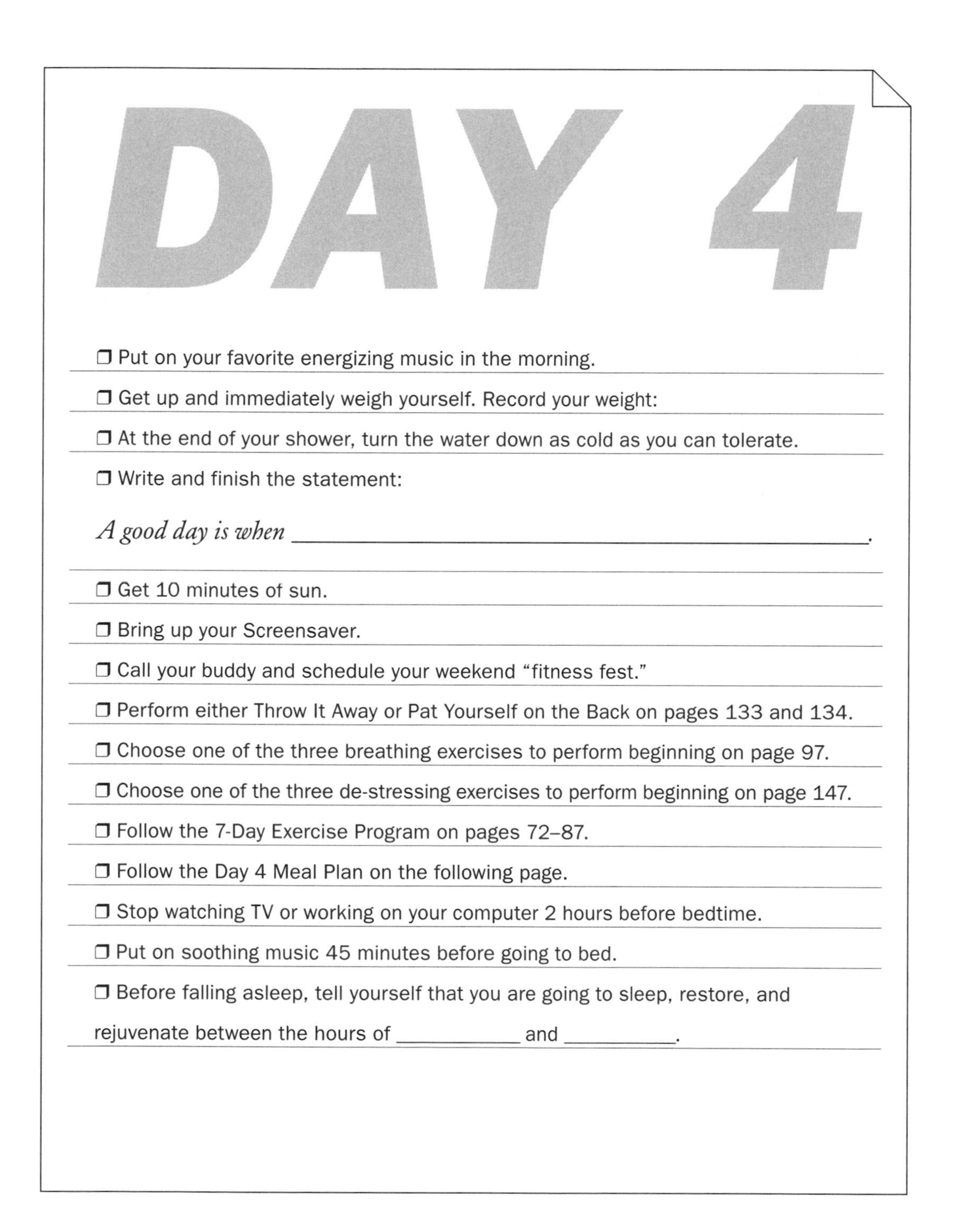

DAY 4

❒ Put on your favorite energizing music in the morning.

❒ Get up and immediately weigh yourself. Record your weight:

❒ At the end of your shower, turn the water down as cold as you can tolerate.

❒ Write and finish the statement:

A good day is when ______________________________________.

❒ Get 10 minutes of sun.

❒ Bring up your Screensaver.

❒ Call your buddy and schedule your weekend "fitness fest."

❒ Perform either Throw It Away or Pat Yourself on the Back on pages 133 and 134.

❒ Choose one of the three breathing exercises to perform beginning on page 97.

❒ Choose one of the three de-stressing exercises to perform beginning on page 147.

❒ Follow the 7-Day Exercise Program on pages 72–87.

❒ Follow the Day 4 Meal Plan on the following page.

❒ Stop watching TV or working on your computer 2 hours before bedtime.

❒ Put on soothing music 45 minutes before going to bed.

❒ Before falling asleep, tell yourself that you are going to sleep, restore, and rejuvenate between the hours of ___________ and __________.

DAY 4

DAY 4 MEAL PLAN
1,240 CALORIES

In addition to the meals below, consume 3 cups of Bieler's Broth, 3+ cups of tea, and no more than 300 milligrams of caffeine in either tea or coffee by noon.

Breakfast — Veggie Scrambled Eggs and Whole Wheat Toast = 216 calories

4 egg whites = 60

½ cup chopped tomato = 19

1 cup chopped red pepper = 26

1 cup chopped broccoli florets = 24

Cooking spray = 7

1 slice whole wheat bread = 80

Combine the egg whites, tomato, red pepper, and broccoli. Coat the inside of a nonstick skillet with cooking spray. Add the mixture to the skillet and cook over medium-high heat until done. Toast the slice of whole wheat bread and eat with the eggs.

Snack — 1 Lärabar = 220 calories

Lunch — Greek Salad with Grilled Salmon = 304 calories

4 ounces skinless poached salmon fillet = 160

3 cups mixed greens = 24

1 ounce feta = 74

½ cup diced cucumber = 7

½ cup chopped tomato = 19

2 tablespoons balsamic vinegar = 20

Grill the salmon until it is opaque throughout and flakes easily with a fork. Combine the greens, feta, cucumber, and tomato in a bowl. Top with the grilled salmon and drizzle with the balsamic vinegar.

Snack — 1 medium-size apple = 87 calories

Dinner — Apple Balsamic Chicken = 312 calories

4 ounces boneless, skinless chicken breast = 192

1 cup diced apple = 64

Salt and pepper

¼ cup balsamic vinegar = 40

2 cups steamed chopped spinach = 16

Preheat the oven to 375°F. Place the chicken in a baking dish and top with the apple. Season with salt and pepper to taste, pour in the balsamic vinegar, and bake until the chicken is opaque throughout. Serve with the steamed spinach.

Snack — 1 large stalk celery and 1 tablespoon peanut butter = 101 calories

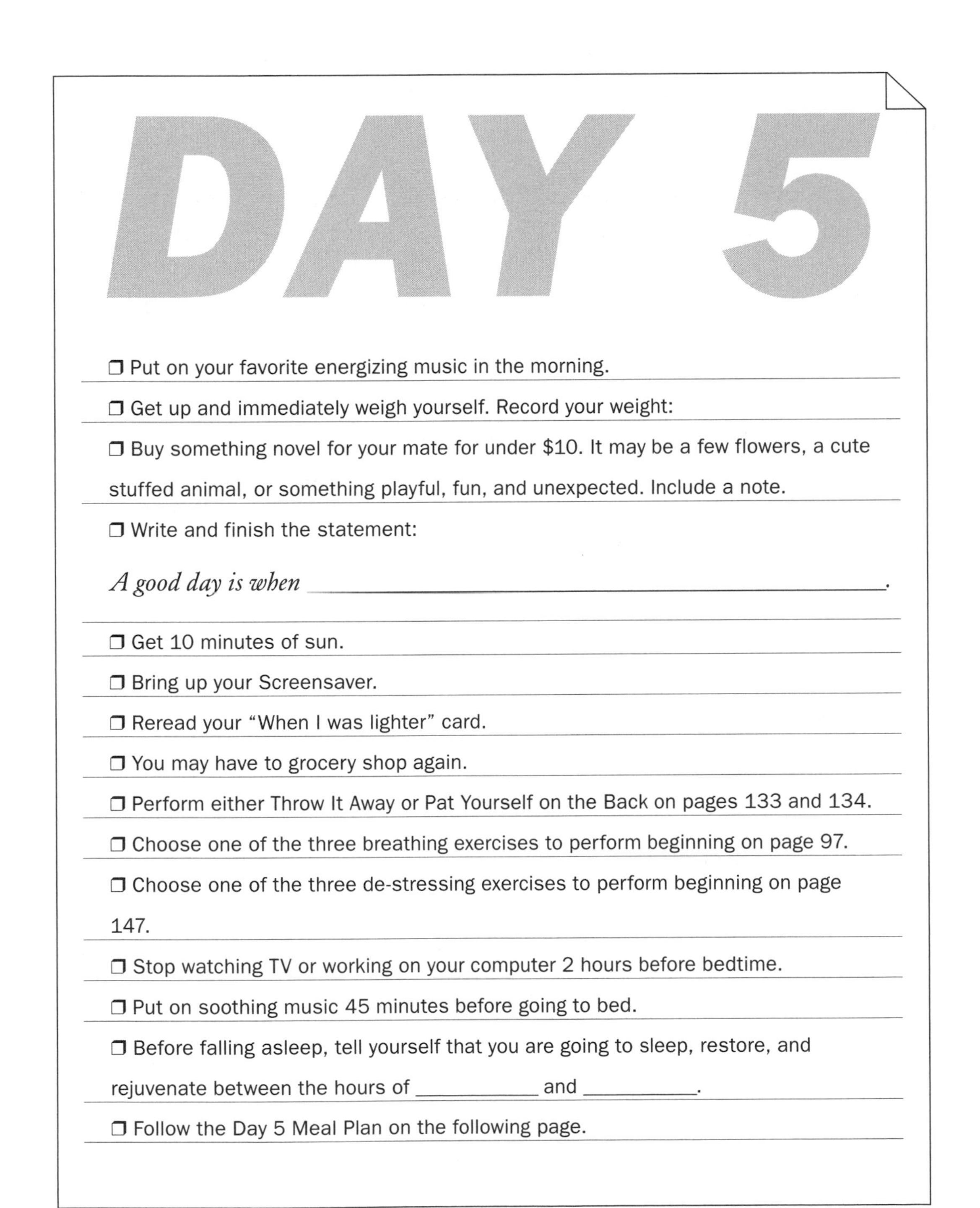

DAY 5

❒ Put on your favorite energizing music in the morning.

❒ Get up and immediately weigh yourself. Record your weight:

❒ Buy something novel for your mate for under $10. It may be a few flowers, a cute stuffed animal, or something playful, fun, and unexpected. Include a note.

❒ Write and finish the statement:

A good day is when ______________________________.

❒ Get 10 minutes of sun.

❒ Bring up your Screensaver.

❒ Reread your "When I was lighter" card.

❒ You may have to grocery shop again.

❒ Perform either Throw It Away or Pat Yourself on the Back on pages 133 and 134.

❒ Choose one of the three breathing exercises to perform beginning on page 97.

❒ Choose one of the three de-stressing exercises to perform beginning on page 147.

❒ Stop watching TV or working on your computer 2 hours before bedtime.

❒ Put on soothing music 45 minutes before going to bed.

❒ Before falling asleep, tell yourself that you are going to sleep, restore, and rejuvenate between the hours of __________ and __________.

❒ Follow the Day 5 Meal Plan on the following page.

DAY
5

DAY 5 MEAL PLAN
1,208 CALORIES

In addition to the meals below, consume 3 cups of Bieler's Broth, 3+ cups of tea, and no more than 300 milligrams of caffeine in either tea or coffee by noon.

Breakfast — Cottage cheese and fruit = 275 calories

½ cup 2% cottage cheese = 90

1 medium-size banana = 105

1 slice whole wheat toast = 80

Combine the cottage cheese and sliced banana in a bowl. Serve with the whole wheat toast.

Snack — String cheese = 80 calories

Lunch — Club Monaco Sandwich = 335 calories

2 slices whole wheat toast = 160

4 slices low-fat turkey = 46

1 hard-boiled egg, sliced = 90

2 lettuce leaves = 3

3 tomato slices = 24

1 tablespoon Dijon mustard = 4

2 pickle spears = 8

Spread the mustard on the toast, and layer the turkey, egg slices, lettuce, and tomato slices on top and serve with the pickles on the side.

Snack — 12 almonds = 91 calories

Dinner — Grilled Tuna with Veggies = 326 calories

6 ounces grilled tuna steak = 246

Salt and pepper

2 tablespoons lemon juice = 8

3 cups broccoli florets, chopped = 72

Season the tuna with salt and pepper. Grill the tuna to your likeness and drizzle with the lemon juice. Steam the broccoli and serve with the tuna.

Snack — 1 large stalk celery and 1 tablespoon peanut butter = 101 calories

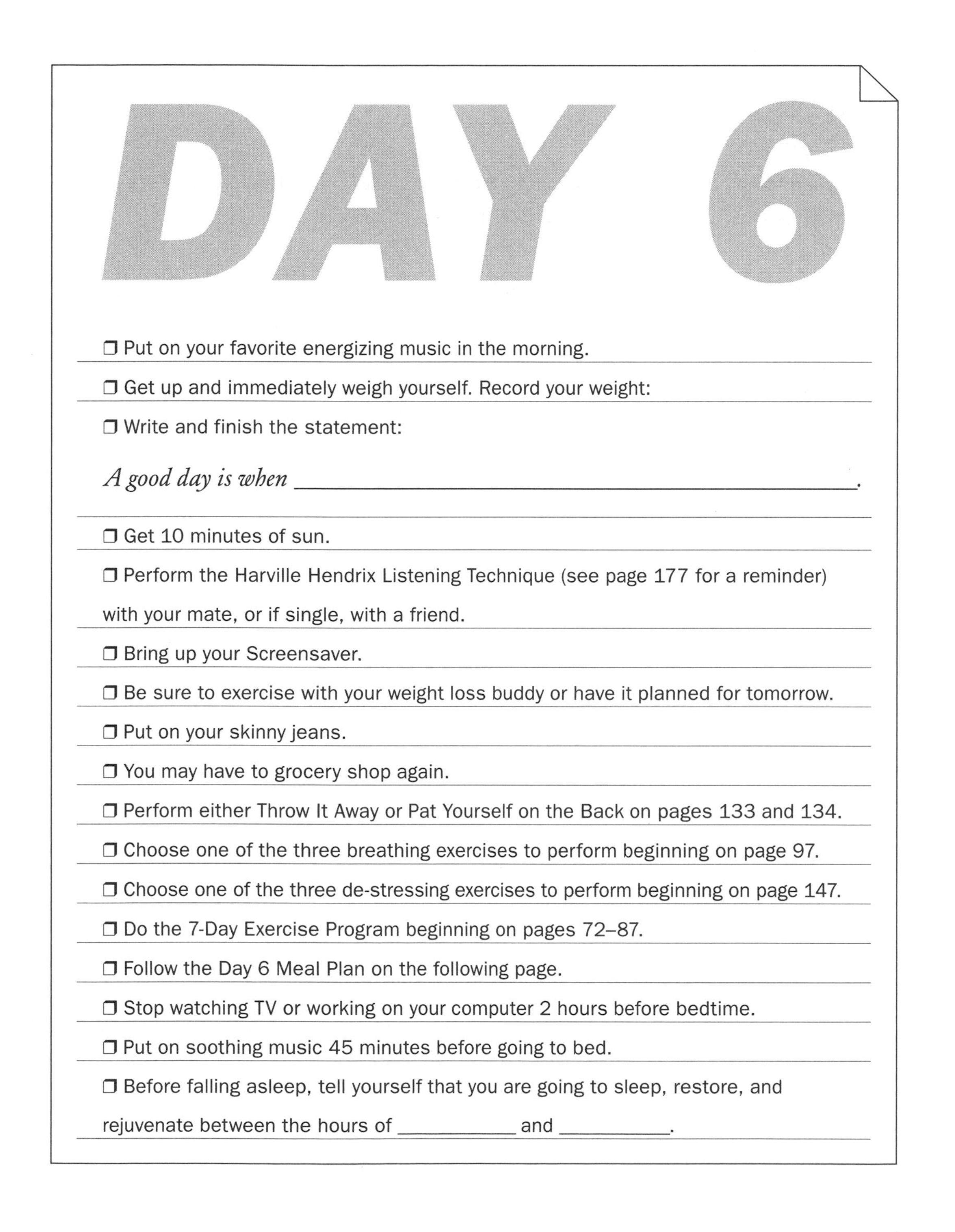

DAY 6

- ❐ Put on your favorite energizing music in the morning.
- ❐ Get up and immediately weigh yourself. Record your weight:
- ❐ Write and finish the statement:

A good day is when ______________________________.

- ❐ Get 10 minutes of sun.
- ❐ Perform the Harville Hendrix Listening Technique (see page 177 for a reminder) with your mate, or if single, with a friend.
- ❐ Bring up your Screensaver.
- ❐ Be sure to exercise with your weight loss buddy or have it planned for tomorrow.
- ❐ Put on your skinny jeans.
- ❐ You may have to grocery shop again.
- ❐ Perform either Throw It Away or Pat Yourself on the Back on pages 133 and 134.
- ❐ Choose one of the three breathing exercises to perform beginning on page 97.
- ❐ Choose one of the three de-stressing exercises to perform beginning on page 147.
- ❐ Do the 7-Day Exercise Program beginning on pages 72–87.
- ❐ Follow the Day 6 Meal Plan on the following page.
- ❐ Stop watching TV or working on your computer 2 hours before bedtime.
- ❐ Put on soothing music 45 minutes before going to bed.
- ❐ Before falling asleep, tell yourself that you are going to sleep, restore, and rejuvenate between the hours of __________ and __________.

DAY 6 MEAL PLAN
1,214 CALORIES

In addition to the meals below, consume 3 cups of Bieler's Broth, 3+ cups of tea, and no more than 300 milligrams of caffeine in either tea or coffee after noon.

Breakfast — Poached eggs, yogurt, and toast = 320 calories

2 eggs = 180

Salt and pepper

Low-fat yogurt = 100

½ slice whole wheat toast = 40

Bring 3 inches of water and the vinegar or lemon juice to a bare simmer in a small pot. Poach the eggs until the whites are set, about 3 minutes, and season with salt and pepper. Serve with the yogurt and toast.

Snack — String cheese = 80 calories

Lunch — Tuna Steak Salad = 325 calories

4 ounces tuna steak = 164

3 cups mixed greens = 24

½ cup diced cucumber = 7

½ cup chopped tomato = 19

12 almonds = 91

2 tablespoons balsamic vinegar = 20

Grill the tuna steak to desired doneness. Combine the greens, cucumber, tomato, and almonds in a bowl. Top with the tuna steak and drizzle with the balsamic vinegar.

Snack — 1 packet oatmeal = 100 calories

Dinner

Shrimp Chili Fajitas = 299 calories

Cooking spray = 7

4 ounces cooked shrimp = 112

1 cup sliced red pepper = 26

¼ cup tomato juice = 10

1 teaspoon chili powder = 8

1 teaspoon garlic powder = 12

2 corn tortillas, warmed = 120

Coat the inside of a large skillet with cooking spray. Add the shrimp and red pepper to a bowl. In a small cup, combine the tomato juice, chili powder, and garlic powder and stir to combine. Pour over the shrimp and toss well. Add to the pan and cook over medium-high heat until the shrimp are cooked through. Put the mixture into the warm tortillas and serve.

Snack

1 medium-size apple = 87 calories

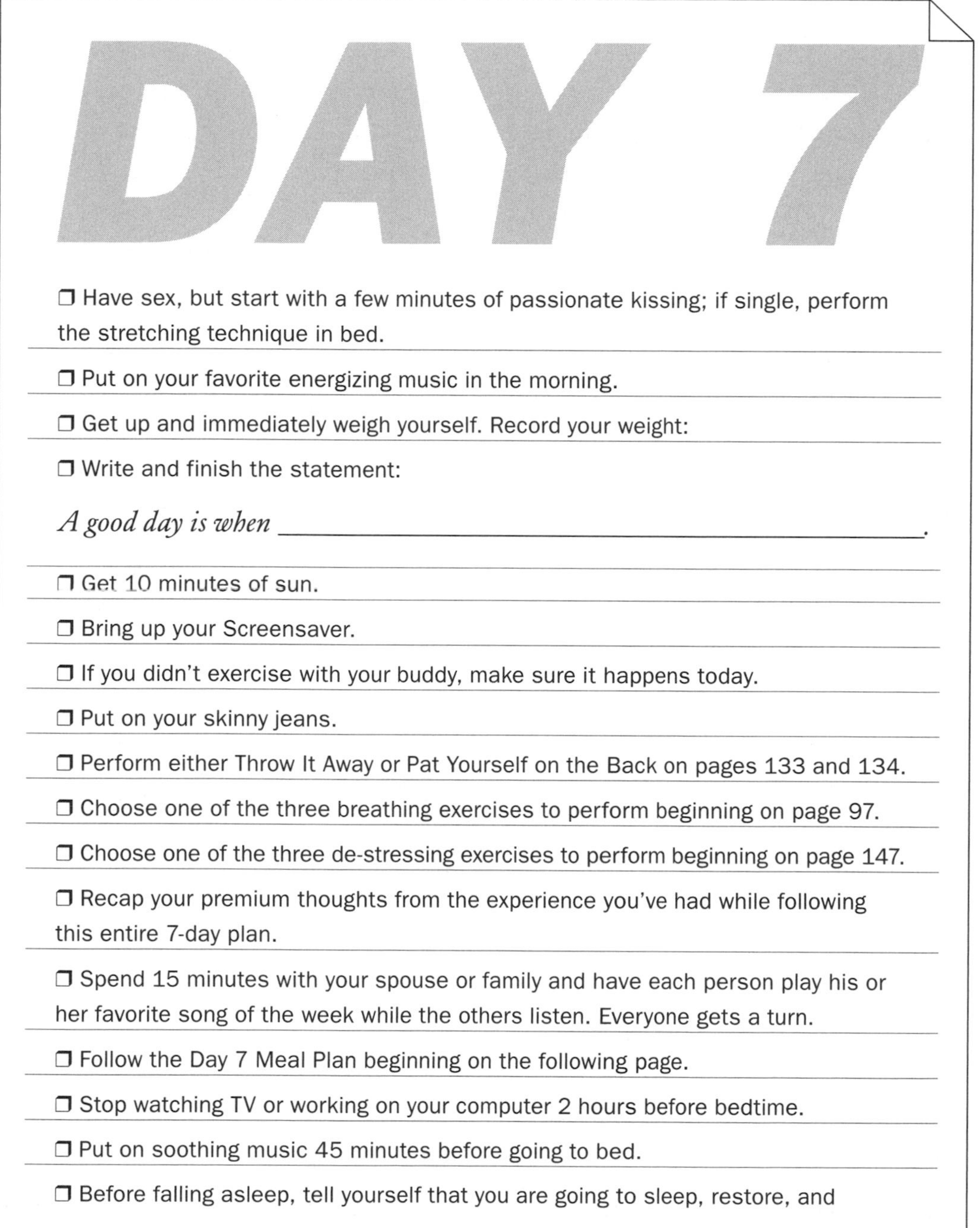

DAY 7

- ❒ Have sex, but start with a few minutes of passionate kissing; if single, perform the stretching technique in bed.
- ❒ Put on your favorite energizing music in the morning.
- ❒ Get up and immediately weigh yourself. Record your weight:
- ❒ Write and finish the statement:

  A good day is when ______________________________.
- ❒ Get 10 minutes of sun.
- ❒ Bring up your Screensaver.
- ❒ If you didn't exercise with your buddy, make sure it happens today.
- ❒ Put on your skinny jeans.
- ❒ Perform either Throw It Away or Pat Yourself on the Back on pages 133 and 134.
- ❒ Choose one of the three breathing exercises to perform beginning on page 97.
- ❒ Choose one of the three de-stressing exercises to perform beginning on page 147.
- ❒ Recap your premium thoughts from the experience you've had while following this entire 7-day plan.
- ❒ Spend 15 minutes with your spouse or family and have each person play his or her favorite song of the week while the others listen. Everyone gets a turn.
- ❒ Follow the Day 7 Meal Plan beginning on the following page.
- ❒ Stop watching TV or working on your computer 2 hours before bedtime.
- ❒ Put on soothing music 45 minutes before going to bed.
- ❒ Before falling asleep, tell yourself that you are going to sleep, restore, and rejuvenate between the hours of __________ and __________.

DAY 7

DAY 7 MEAL PLAN
1,218 CALORIES

In addition to the meals below, consume 3 cups of Bieler's Broth, 3+ cups of tea, and no more than 300 milligrams of caffeine in either tea or coffee by noon.

Breakfast — Breakfast Burrito = 291 calories

Cooking spray = 7

4 egg whites = 60

1 cup sliced red pepper = 26

½ cup chopped tomato = 19

1 slice Sargento reduced-fat Cheddar = 60

2 corn tortillas = 120

Coat the inside of a nonstick skillet with cooking spray. Mix the egg whites, pepper, and tomato in a bowl and add to the pan. Scramble until fully cooked. Cut the slice of cheese in half, place each piece on a tortilla, and serve with the scrambled eggs.

Snack — Low-fat yogurt = 100 calories

Lunch — Apple Almond Crunch Salad with Shrimp = 320 calories

Cooking spray = 7

4 ounces cooked shrimp = 112

3 cups mixed greens = 24

1 cup chopped cucumber = 14

12 almonds = 91

1 cup sliced apple = 64

¼ cup sliced red onion = 15

2 tablespoons balsamic vinegar = 20

Coat the inside of a nonstick skillet with cooking spray. Sauté the shrimp over medium heat until opaque throughout. Combine the greens, cucumber, almonds, sliced apple, red onion, and cooked shrimp in a bowl and serve.

Snack — 1 large stalk celery and 1 tablespoon peanut butter = 101 calories

Dinner — Lemon Chicken = 296 calories

5 ounces boneless, skinless chicken breast = 240

2 tablespoons lemon juice = 8

Salt and pepper

2 cups broccoli florets, chopped = 48

Preheat the oven to 350°F. In a small ovenproof dish, place the chicken, drizzle with lemon juice, and season with salt and pepper. Bake for 30 minutes, or until cooked through and opaque. Steam the broccoli to desired doneness and serve with the chicken.

Snack — ½ cup 2% cottage cheese = 90 calories

CONCLUSION

KEEPING THE SURGE

Now that you have completed your 7-Day Energy Surge, you need to retake the 7-Day Energy Surge Quiz (page xvi) and assess which variables you have successfully mastered, which variables need more of your attention, and which variables you might have avoided. I hope you were able to successfully improve your score. *Note:* Take this test again in the future because it will be motivating to have measurable results in front of you.

Now, we all gravitate to what is easy, familiar, and within our comfort zone and avoid the rest. If stress is a major issue, then you need to spend more time on the techniques and tools Cynthia and I introduced to you. Repetition is the key to success. If you don't believe me, then read what two relatively bright guys have to say about it:

"We are what we repeatedly do—Excellence, therefore, is not an act but a habit."—Aristotle

"Repetition of the same thought or physical action develops into a habit, which, repeated frequently enough, becomes an automatic reflex."—Norman Vincent Peale

Make it a new habit *not* to avoid issues as you have done in the past; be proactive and take control. Back in the introduction, I stated that increased energy is truly one of the most intoxicating, natural experiences I have ever had and now *you* have the skills and knowledge to create it as well. It's your life. No one is going to do it for you; you've got to put yourself first.

Let's stick with that for a moment; consider your needs an important priority. I know that sounds selfish, but I firmly believe that selfish, in the right context, is *good* and bumps up your energy *and* your energy field. Everyone benefits.

Say you are a stay-at-home mom; where do your needs lie in the pecking order we call life? I bet it's kids, husband, home, shopping, cooking, cleaning, chauffeuring, scheduling, and on and on. Where do you fall in that order? Rock bottom. That makes NO sense. You would be a far better mother, spouse, and friend if you were in better shape, ate and drank the right things, got much-needed exercise and sleep, breathed, cleared your mind, decreased stress, listened to music, and made it essential that you and your mate spend much-needed alone time. When you move up on that list, EVERYONE benefits; it's a win-win situation.

Ditto for the stressed, overworked executive. It's work, work, work, then maybe a little time for friends or family, and that's it. Can you even remember that last time you had sex? You probably feel like crap, probably are starting to look like crap, and exist by eating and drinking, well . . . crap. The moment you put your foot down and spend just a few minutes a day on you, your creativity, productivity, memory, appearance, patience–everything else–will soar. You might even get lucky!

After you have completed this 7-Day Energy Surge, please realize that life is going to continually present unforeseen challenges, such as a demanding boss, difficulty in your marriage or primary relationship, managing the "terrible twos" through the "troubling teens," illness, death, and a host of other obstacles. When one of these life-changing events strikes, most people toss their new "energy-positive" habits and fall back into "energy-destructive" ones. Make this time different, and together let's devise a strategy to make it through the rough times without annihilating your newfound, productive energy.

ENERGY IN DANGEROUS TERRITORY

Life is constantly taking us to unfamiliar places, or familiar places that routinely present a challenge. Here are some tips on how to stay on track and energized to meet those challenges.

Traveling, for Business or Pleasure

What is it about travel that causes all good judgment to go "on holiday"? These days, we travel for work, family, pleasure, you name it, and we must be prepared for the worst. Here is what I advise:

- Pack the right snacks. Do not get on an airplane, a train, or even into your car without a few boxes of raisins, some energy bars (just watch the calorie count), nuts, or apples, or know that the airport or station has a vendor with the right choices.
- Schedule your workouts. These are very important. Make a plan, then follow through with the plan. Remember the quotation "A failure to plan is a plan to fail."

- Watch your alcohol consumption. For most people, when "booze" is around, all good judgment flies out the window.
- Schedule travel intelligently. DON'T take the last flight out for an early morning meeting, only to discover that it is seriously delayed or even cancelled. That will stress you out and decimate your energy. Also, leave at a time in the morning that allows you to get a full night's sleep.

Managing the Holidays

I don't just mean the holidays between Thanksgiving and New Year's, I mean all of them, when family, friends, food, and drink are concerned. Follow these guidelines:

1. Go to bed early the night before and sleep in. That's why they're called "holidays," and even though I urged you to keep consistent sleep/wake patterns, there are a few days that you may make an exception. This is one of them.

2. Get up and eat one of the breakfast options on the 7-Day Energy Surge.

3. Perform interval strength training.

4. Eat one of the lunches from the 7-Day Energy Surge.

5. Guzzle water–preferably cold, sparkling water.

6. Practice one or all of your stress-reducing techniques because, let's face it, holidays equal stress.

7. Listen to soothing music on the way over, if you're headed to a friend or family member's home, or as you're cleaning and preparing for guests.

8. Waltz into the event with full-belly breathing.

9. Make sure that a big steamed vegetable dish will be a part of the dinner or offer to bring one.

10. Schedule a speedy departure if being around the family pops "issues" and causes you to fall into energy-depleting patterns.

11. Don't make this a caloric/energy disaster, and remember that Thanksgiving Day (or whichever holiday you happen to be celebrating) is just a "day" and not your downfall. Don't start a 4-day domino-eating frenzy, as you have in the past.

Entertaining or Being Entertained

If within your control, choose the right restaurant. Everyone talks about how hard it is to eat out. I *totally* disagree. Sure, it can be a challenge, but *many things in life* are a challenge, and you either choose to accept it or choose to let the challenge devour your energy. I'm not expecting you to live a monastic experience, but the "taste" of energy will far outweigh the taste of buffalo wings with Roquefort dressing if you give it a chance. When eating out, here are a few guidelines:

1. Ask for the breadbasket to be taken away (or not brought in the first place). I know it's free, I know it's habitual, but by passing on the bread you just won round 1 for energy.

2. Ready to win round 2? Take a look at this box, which gives you the do's and don'ts for each different type of restaurant:

Steakhouse	Do order a shrimp cocktail, an 8-ounce filet, a plain baked potato with chives, and a large steamed vegetable. Don't eat the fried calamari, order a 27-ounce Porterhouse steak, load your potato with bacon bits, butter, and sour cream, and finish this off with a big piece of cheesecake.
Italian	Do start with a salad with dressing on the side (and not a Caesar), then have grilled fish (with very little oil), a large steamed vegetable, and some polenta, which is baked cornmeal. Don't order the oil-ridden antipasto platter, the pasta, anything fried, and please, skip the cannolis!
Mexican	Do start with a salad topped with just salsa (it's great), then have chicken, beef, or shrimp fajitas done in very little oil, corn tortillas, and even more salsa. Don't eat any of the rice or beans (hugely full of fat), the guacamole (ditto), the burrito (you have no clue how many calories are wrapped up in there), and the gigantic margarita. Tip: Order some tequila on the rocks and sip.
Chinese	Do order steamed vegetables with chicken, beef, or shrimp and brown rice, and drizzle some low-sodium soy sauce on top. Don't order Kung Pao Chicken, which could add up to thousands of calories, spring rolls (they're fried), or anything saucy.

Thai	Do order soft-wrapped spring or summer rolls with vegetables or shrimp, then have steamed or grilled fish with spices and brown rice. Don't order Pad Thai (the most popular dish, which is thousands of calories), mild coconut curries, or any options with lots of sauce.
French	Do order beet and goat cheese salad with dressing on the side, then order grilled salmon with lentils and chopped vegetables or baked chicken (just get rid of the skin). Don't eat the butter-laden escargot, the steak frites, the fat-filled duck, or anything in a casserole dish.
Sushi	Do order the edamame, cucumber or tuna rolls (*not* spicy tuna, because "spicy" means mayonnaise, which means lots of calories), and six pieces of classic sushi or sashimi. Don't order tempura (a true energy annihilator) or anything fried, overdo the soy and teriyaki sauce, or eat the green tea ice cream. It may sound healthy, but it's not!

The Dreaded Dinner Party . . .

. . . and You Are the Host

Even the smallest gathering comes with a certain amount of stress: Your home needs to be cleaned; you have to plan, shop, then prepare the food; there has to be enough to drink; and you have to be attentive to each of your guests' needs. Start with cheese, grapes, pears, and some low-calorie crackers. Then, plan a healthy meal with sauces on the side. Serve your salad very lightly dressed. You can't go wrong with most things poached–poached salmon is easy and delicious. Then serve both a tasty dessert and fresh fruit. Done. It doesn't need to be an energy-debilitating disaster.

. . . and You Are the Guest

The worst is being a culinary/social prisoner at a dinner party, because your host and/or hostess is watching you eat. If you can, diplomatically ask what is being served for dinner, because you may have to eat before and just pick at the dinner and ask whether you can have any sauces served on the side. Watch your drinking, because each glass adds calories *and* the likelihood that you will lose your resolve. Take the dessert, take a bite, gush to your host or hostess, and call it a day. If all else fails, make nice with the dog!

At a big party with passed hors d'oeuvres and a buffet, only eat the fresh shrimp (most other choices are a caloric nightmare). Fully peruse the buffet before making your selections, choose the smallest plate, start with vegetables, yada, yada, yada.

Dealing with a BAD Influence, Whether Family Member, Friend, or Foe

Do you know a person who totally sucks the energy from you? I can name a few, and I try my very best to avoid them. Some people are simply toxic, so listen to your warning signs when you are feeling drained of your precious energy.

Friendships have a powerful impact on our lives, affecting all areas, from health, career, and relationships to families, children, and aging. When the balance between friends is lacking and one person is giving a lot more than receiving, the friendship becomes toxic, draining, suffocating, unsupportive, and unrewarding.

A circle of friends is essential to a full, rich, balanced life and to supportive energy. It's the family you build; the one you never had, but dreamed of. When assessing each of your friendships, ask:

- Who drains you emotionally, financially, or physically?
- Who is critical of you?
- Who do you dread seeing?
- Who do you come away from feeling accepted and cherished and with renewed, boundless energy?

The Dark Force

Unfortunately, in life, there are many dark forces you can't ignore, and many come in the guise of the human form. It would be nice if we could just avoid and not have to deal with these people. But what should you do when the energy vampire comes in the form of a family member, co-worker, or boss?

- **Family member–Keep interaction to a minimum.** Just because the person is a family member doesn't mean he has to be privy to the facts of your life. Stick to conversations revolving around food, shopping, entertainment, and travel. If your current relationship resembles the *War of the Roses* and this family member asks how it's going, memorize this response: "Everything is going as it should be. I'm SOOOOO happy. Life couldn't be better." Remember, the best revenge is living well.
- **Co-worker.** The all-too-familiar, backstabbing co-worker is a true reality in life. So become the greatest strategist around. Sicken her with saccharine sweetness, keep 10

steps ahead of her game plan, or don't let her know you are on to her. The key is to develop a protective, psychic outer coating. Look at this person and see just how miserable she must be in her life, don't take it personally, and allow her words and actions to slip off of you.

- **Boss.** This is a tough one, because this person has to be tolerated, outwardly respected, and managed. If it is unbearable, spruce up your resume, make some inquiries, and put out some feelers. In the meantime, don't forget your stress management techniques of breathing, meditation, and music. Try to kill the boss with kindness and patience and you may emerge victorious. If you do get slammed by "Bosszilla," use a "lifeline," "phone a friend," and hitch a ride back to your upward "life spiral."

What to Do in a Dangerous Situation

There is nothing worse than getting stuck in the wrong place, with the wrong food, and, most likely, the wrong attitude. Here's what you need to do:

- **Go to the bathroom or a quiet place and give yourself a little pep talk.** At the very least, breathe!
- **If it helps, right there perform one (or more) of the breathing, mind-set, or de-stressing exercises.** Many of these can be done without anyone noticing. Throw It Away may come in really handy. *Note:* I like to use physicality to de-stress. Just saying "calm down" or "you can get through this" isn't as effective for me as thinking, saying, and then physically moving to discharge the tension.
- **Look at your options.** If stuck at a Mexican buffet filled with chips, guacamole, cheese, and more, take a corn tortilla, add lettuce and tomato from the taco bar, and cover it with salsa and some of the beef or chicken. And do a quick Mexican hat dance out the door before the dulce de leche hits the table. Done.
- **Hum your favorite soothing tune.** A lot of people sing or hum in the bathroom, so don't be shy. "Don't Worry, Be Happy" may do the trick.
- **Quickly recall the last funny TV show or movie that made you laugh out loud.** Remember, just anticipating the laugh changes internal chemistry.
- **Bring up your Screensaver.**

- **Be creative.** Resist throwing in the towel and your energy. There has to be some way to salvage the situation. You can always resort to actively kissing your date or fellow party guest.

ADVANCED ENERGY-ENHANCING TECHNIQUES

Connect with Others

We all know and have experienced the impact of other people's energy, be it positive or negative, on our psyche. If you find yourself laughing, feeling comfortable and accepted, and being highly entertained in the presence of another, spend more time cultivating that relationship. Text, call, or e-mail this person or persons right now to give yourself more of that energy connection high. Remember, just anticipating spending time with this person will give you an immediate bump. Throughout your days, be open to how many connections you can make. Some of my greatest connections have been in the wee hours of the morning in a taxicab with a stranger when I ask, "How's life?" Be an energy conduit between you, others, and the world.

Create Something

As discussed earlier, doing different and unfamiliar activities or pursuits expands, restructures, and stimulates the brain. A few months ago, I brought home a puzzle that was a challenge for my kids and me. We became obsessed with finishing the puzzle and would applaud each other when we got a piece and praise each other for the good work; my home bubbled with excitement as we were pushing for the end goal. Whether it's an enticing recipe, a model airplane, the building blocks of a new language, a CD mix, a challenging yoga pose, or creating ambience for when your mate or friends come over, stretch yourself, push yourself, and always reach for the novel and new.

Energize Your Spiritual Life

My good friend Peggy urged me not to minimize the power of faith, whether it be through organized religion and attending services or through your own spiritual rituals that ground you and give you hope, peace of mind, and happiness. All of those things are going to be energy "uppers," and if you don't believe me, then look at the faces of many people after they have attended a religious service. A study reported by the National Institute on Aging found that people who regularly attended church, synagogue, mosque, or temple reduced the risk of early death by 35 percent for women and 17 percent for men.[1] The researchers aren't even sure why this was the case, but they speculated that regular attendance led to less stress, depression, and anxiety; that the behavior of those who attend religious services is generally healthier than that of nonattendees; and that regular attendance created the very powerful effects of social connection.

Now, for those of you who don't find organized religious services to be energy additive, you too have options. There are many organizations that possess a strong spiritual component but don't include strict rules and religious dogma. One that comes to mind is the Self-Realization Fellowship, which has locations all over the country. Or you might consider volunteering; many studies have shown that volunteer work promotes "happiness, life satisfaction, self-esteem, sense of control over life and physical health."[2] Volunteers are needed now more than ever in these difficult, sometimes frightening times.

As you can see, this book is not about the perfect body, the "only be positive" mind-set, or übersex. It is a holistic book of knowledge for developing your mind, body, and soul. Use it with gusto. Dive in headfirst and come out vibrating with the *energy* of possibility.

The earth has an electrical field, the sun and moon a gravitational pull; energy exists everywhere in nature and affects us in marvelous ways. Just visualize a beautiful sunset, hear the roar of the ocean, smell the cookies in the oven. Energy also affects us in not so marvelous ways–natural disasters, war, and poverty, to name a few. Each and every one of our positive and negative thoughts and behaviors has an effect on the earth as well as on each other, and some of these events have taken years to transpire.

We are facing an overwhelming energy crisis in this country, but we are focusing on the energy needed to eat, stay warm or cool, or travel from one place to another. Let's face it, there is only so much you can do to conserve this form of energy, but there are infinite changes you can and should make to increase your prized, life-altering energy.

Change can occur in an instant, if you work at it, accept it, refine it, and welcome it. You can't buy energy in a store, but you *are* in control of nurturing and enhancing your own precious, potent, potential energy, and this book should be your first step in reclaiming your *capacity of a physical system to do work.*

Now optimize that system by how you eat, drink, move, breathe, sleep, think, and deal with stress . . . then add music . . . and whom you touch in *many* ways. Surprise yourself and inspire others.

Good luck!

ENDNOTES

Component 1: Body Weight to Surge

1. F. Wang, "Association of Healthcare Costs with Per Unit Body Mass Index Increase," *Journal of Occupational and Environmental Medicine* 48, no. 7 (2006): 668–74.
2. Healthy News Service, "Weight Loss Significantly Improves Sexual Quality of Life," http://www.healthy.net/scr/news.asp?Id=7971.
3. R. Wing et al, "A Self-Regulation Program for Maintenance of Weight Loss," *New England Journal of Medicine* 15, no. 355 (2006): 1563–71.
4. L. Grieger, "Weighing In," http://yourtotalhealth.ivillage.com/diet-fitness/weighing-in.html.
5. Helen Croker and Lyndel Costain, "Helping Individuals to Help Themselves," *American Journal of Clinical Nutrition* 64 (2005): 1189–96.
6. A. Paturel, "The ABCs of Slim," *Women's Health* (January-February 2008): 104.
7. Elizabeth M. Ward, "Research Uncovers Dramatic New Health Roles for Vitamin D," *Environmental Nutrition* 27, no. 4 (2004): 1–4.

Component 2: Eat to Surge

1. Liz Plosser, "8 Things You Always Wanted to Know about Dieting," http://www.webmd.com/diet/features/know-about-dieting-who-ask?.
2. N. Hellmich, "Got Milk–and Got Controversy," *USA Today* (March 9, 2006): 5.
3. Ibid.
4. "Which Fruits and Vegetables Are the Most Toxic?" *Best Life* (August 2008): 22.
5. N. Hellmich, "Apple a Day Keeps the Calories at Bay," *USA Today* (October 23, 2007): 32.
6. "About That Apple a Day," *Men's Health* (July-August 2008): 42.
7. "Apples Prevent Mammary Tumors in Rats," *Journal of Agriculture and Food Chemistry* 53 (6) (March 23, 2005): 2341–43.
8. "Wellness Facts," *Wellness Letter* 24, no. 6 (March 2008): 1.
9. *Tufts University Health & Nutrition Letter* (May 2008): 6.
10. *Tufts University Health & Nutrition Letter* (December 2007): 8.
11. "A Dream Diet," *Men's Health* (July-August 2008): 46.
12. Haidong Kan, June Stevens, Gerardo Heiss, Kathryn M. Rose, and Stephanie J. London, *American Journal of Epidemiology* 167, Issue 5 (March 2008): 570–578.
13. Shape.com, "8 Things You Always Wanted to Know About Dieting," http://www.shape.com/healthy_eating/articles/dieting_myths.html?page=4.
14. J. Ivy, "Timing Is Everything," University of Texas at Austin, http://www.utexas.edu/features/archive/2004/nutrition.html.
15. A. Cunliffe, "The Role of Diet and Exercise," *Asia Pacific Journal of Clinical Nutrition* 10, no. 3 (2006): 226–32.
16. "Rev Your Metabolism," *Best Life* (August 2008): 58.
17. Mayoclinic.com, "Weight Loss: 6 Strategies for Success," http://www.mayoclinic.com/heath/weight-loss/HQ01625.
18. "Use Your Nose to Stay Trim," *Best Life* (October 2008): 66.
19. "Why Go Nuts," *University of California, Berkeley Wellness Letter* 24, no. 8 (May 2008): 1–2.

20. Elizabeth Ward, "How Breakfast Can Help You Lose Weight, Even Stave Off Disease," *Environmental Nutrition* (September 2003), http://findarticles.com/p/articles/mi_m0854/is_9_26/ai_n18616249.

21. Henry Legere, *Raising Healthy Eaters: 100 Tips for Parents* (Cambridge, MA: Da Capo Press, 2004), 69.

22. Ibid.

23. Karen Ansel, "Your 3-Step Plan to Trim Extra Calories without Counting, Dieting, or Feeling Deprived," *Prevention* (January 2008): 149.

24. "Solving the Portion Puzzle," *Tufts University Health & Nutrition Letter* (December 2007): 4–5.

25. C. Martins, L. Morgan, and H. Truby, "A Review of the Effects of Exercise on Appetite Regulation: An Obesity Perspective," *International Journal of Obesity* 32, no. 9 (September 2008): 1337–47.

26. Brian Wansink and Pierre Chandon, "Meal Size, Not Body Size, Explains Errors in Estimating the Calorie Content of Meals," *Annals of Internal Medicine* 145, no. 5 (September 2006): 326–332.

27. S. Kechagias, Å. Ernersson, O. Dahlqvist, P. Lundberg, T. Lindström, and F. H. Nystrom, "Fast-Food-Based Hyper-alimentation Can Induce Rapid and Profound Elevation of Serum Alanine Aminotransferase in Healthy Subjects," *Gut Journal* 57 (May 2008): 649–54.

Component 3: Drink to Surge

1. Janet Helm, "Think Before You Drink: Watch Out for Covert Calories in Beverages," *Environmental Nutrition* 31, no. 4 (April 2008): 1, 6.

2. Med Journal Watch, "Avoid Liquid Calories," http://medjournalwatch.blogspot.com/2007/07/avoid-liquid-calories.html (July 2, 2007).

3.Myatt Murphy, "Live the Fat Burning Life," WebMD, http://www.webmd.com/diet/features/live-fat-burning-life?

4. Judelson, A., et al. "Effect of Hydration State on Resistance Exercise-Induced Endocrine Markers of Anabolism, Catabolism, and Metabolism," *Journal of Applied Physiology.* (September 10, 2008):816–24

5. Selene Yeager, "High-Metabolism Diet: Essential Eating Rules That Stoke Your Fat Burn All Day Long," *Prevention* (March 2008): 138.

6. "Water Works," *Men's Health* (March 2008): 54.

7. "Diet Now–Ice Burner," *Health Magazine* (June 2008): 20.

8. "Lose Weight with Sparkling Water," *Best Life* (September 2008): 82.

9. "Boil It Down," *Men's Health* (December 2005): 52.

10. "Your Cup of Tea," *Men's Health* (March 2004): 48.

11. "Drink This, Go Long," *Men's Health* (June 2005): 56.

12. "The Best New Drink for Lifters," *Men's Health* (June 2008): 62.

13. Jeffrey Blumberg, "Introduction to the Proceedings of the Third International Scientific Symposium on Tea and Human Health: Role of Flavonoids in the Diet," *Journal of Nutrition,* (October 2003), Vol. 133, issue 10, 3244-3246

14. Rosemary Ellis, "Tea totalling," *Town & Country* (June 2003): 132.

15. PRNewswire "New Research Provides Evidence That Tea May Improve Attention and Focus."

16. "Brewing Up Health Benefits for Coffee," *Tufts University Health & Nutrition Letter* (January 2008): 4–5.

17. Lauren Griffin, "The Caffeine Advantage," *Men's Health* (March 2008): 104.

18. Ibid.

19. Ilango Karuppannan, "12 Tips for a Fat Burning Diet," http://ezinearticles.com/?12-Tips-for-a-Fat-Burning-Diet&id=1003247.

20. Angela Haupt, "Coffee May Have Perks for Longer Living," *USA Today*, June 16, 2008.

21. "Brewing Up Health Benefits for Coffee," *Tufts University Health & Nutrition Letter* (January 2008): 4–5.

22. Caroline Wilbert, "Most Who Have Prediabetes Don't Know It," http://diabetes.webmd.com/news/20081106/most-have-prediabetes-don't-know-it (November 6, 2008).
23. Harvard School of Public Health Press Release, "Long-Term Coffee Consumption Linked to Reduced Risk for Type 2 Diabetes," http://www.hsph.harvard.edu/news/press-releases/archives/2004 (January 5, 2004).
24. "Coffee May Reduce Liver Cancer Risk," *New Scientist Magazine*, no. 2488 (February 26, 2005): 21.
25. Nescafe.com, "Coffee May Reduce Colon Cancer Risk Among Women," http://www.nescafe.com/NR/rdonlyres/4AA5B93F-1E25-4099-A8AF-AE106170241E/84531/CoffeeAug07ColonCancer.pdf.
26. "Caffeine Reduces Risk of Parkinson's," *Harvard University Gazette* (May 10, 2001): 10–12.
27. AGA News Release, "Harvard Nurses' Health Study: Coffee Lowers Risk of Gallstone Disease in Women," http://www.gastro.org/wmspage.cfm?parm1+429.
28. "Caffeine for Smooth Skin," *Best Life* (August 2008): 56.
29. Miranda Hitti, "Coffee May Raise Heart Disease Risk: Moderate Amounts Raise Inflammation and May Increase Risk, Says Greek Study," WebMD (October 2004), http://www.webmd.com/heart-disease/news/20041020/coffee-may-raise-heart-disease-risk.
30. Kathleen Doheny, "Milk: The Best Muscle-Builder?" MedicineNet.com (August 2007), http://medicinenet.com/script/main/art.asp?articlekey=83113.
31. "Alcohol and Breast Cancer," *University of California, Berkeley Wellness Letter* 24, issue 5 (February 2008): 3.
32. "Is Alcohol Still Safe in Moderation?" *Healthy Living* (July 2008): 3.
33. Amy Z. Fan, Marcia Russell, et al, "Associations of Lifetime Alcohol Drinking Trajectories with Cardiometabolic Risk," *Journal of Clinical Endocrinology and Metabolism* 93, no. 1 (2008): 154–61.
34. Stephanie Breakstone, "Newest Soda Danger: The Pop Belly," *Prevention* (July 2008): 68.
35. Lisa Conti, "Faux Sugar: Bittersweet," *Scientific American Mind* (June-July 2008): 14.
36. Harvard School of Public Health Press Release, "Study Finds Increased Consumption of Sugar-Sweetened Beverages Promotes Childhood Obesity," http://www.hsph.harvard.edu/new/press-releases/archives/2001-releases (February 15, 2001).

Component 4: Exercise to Surge

1. Michael Stefano, "When It Comes to Exercise, Less Is More," Seekwellness.com, http://seekwellness.com/fitness/less_is_more.html.
2. Rochelle L. Goldsmith et al, "Implementation of a Novel Cyclic Exercise Protocol in Healthy Women," *American Journal of Medicine* 4, no. 2 (March-April 2002): 135–41.
3. "Go Heavy to Get Light," *Men's Health* (March 2006): 54.
4. Alwyn Cosgrove, "The Hierarchy of Fat Loss," www.alwyncosgrove.com/hierarchy-of-fat-loss.html.
5. Phil Campbell, "Walk (or Run) This Way," *O: The Oprah Magazine* (September 2007): 228.
6. Jade Teta and Keoni Teta, "The 3 Mechanisms That Burn Belly Fat," *OnFitness Magazine* 9, no. 2 (2008): 32.
7. "Strength Training Reduces Neck Pain in Women," *Fitness Journal* (April 2008): 14.
8. "The End of the Iron Age," *Men's Health* (July-August 2008): 36.
9. Ibid.
10. "Instant Energy," *Men's Health* (September 2008): 56.
11. Mark Moyad, "Age Erasers: The Science of Staying Young," *Best Life* (May 2008): 24–28
12. "Strength Gain Showdown: Fixed vs. Freeform Equipment," *Fitness Journal* (April 2008): 16.
13. "Standing Room Only," *Women's Health* (May 2008): 26.
14. Judith Norkin, "Exercise: A Radical Proposition," *Life Extension Magazine* (September 1998): 1–3.

15. Alwyn Cosgrove, "The Hierarchy of Fat Loss," op cit, no. 4, above.
16. Charles Poliquin, "Six Reasons Why Aerobic Work Is Counterproductive," http://www.charlespoliquin.com/index.php?option=com_content&task=view&id=861.
17. M. Van Middelkoop, J. Kolkman, J. Van Ochten, S. M. A. Bierma-Zeinstra, and B. Koes, "Prevalence and Incidence of Lower Extremity Injuries in Male Marathon Runners," *Scandinavian Journal of Medicine and Science in Sports* 18, no. 2 (April 2008): 140–44.
18. "Switch on Your Six-Pack," *Men's Health* (July-August 2008): 52.
19. Elizabeth Quinn, "Midday Exercise Improves Employee Productivity," http://sportsmedicine.about.com/od/tipsandtricks/a/midday_exercise.htm (July 19, 2006).
20. "The Excuse I'm Too Tired to Work Out," *Women's Health* (May 2008): 36.

Component 5: Breathe to Surge

1. Judith Anodea, Llewellyn Worldwide (1999): 214.
2. Todd Zwillich, "High Carbon Dioxide Levels May Up Asthma Rate," WebMD, http://www.webmd.com/asthma/news/20040429/high-carbon-dioxide-levels-may-up-asthma-rate (April 29, 2004).
3. S. Elliott and D. Edmonson, *The New Science of Breath: Coherent Breathing for Autonomic Nervous System Balance, Health, and Well-being* (Allen, TX: Coherence Publishing, 2005), 67–138.
4. Gay Hendricks, *Conscious Breathing* (New York: Bantam Dell, 1995), 16–17.
5. Jack Shield, "Lymph Glands and Homeostasis," *Lymphology* 25, no. 4 (December 1992): 147–153.
6. Ali Majid, *Oxygen and Aging* (Denville, NJ: Canary Press, 2003), 192.
7. B. Kangae Lee, Robert A. Roth, and John J. LaPres, "Hypoxia, Drug Therapy, and Toxicity," *Pharmacology & Therapeutics* 113, no. 2 (February 2007): 229–246.
8. S. Toffoli and C. Michiels, "Intermittent Hypoxia Is a Key Regulator of Cancer Cell and Endothelial Cell Interplay in Tumours," *FEBS Journal* 275, no. 12 (June 2008): 2991–3002.
9. Jan Dixhoorn and Adrian White, "Relaxation Therapy for Rehabilitation and Prevention in Ischaemic Heart Disease," *Journal of Psychosomatic Research* 61 (2006): 1–7.
10. "How Much Stress Does It Take to Make a Man Go Grey?" *Best Life* (October 2008): 20.
11. David Schipper, "Outsmart Your Stomach," *Men's Health* (October 2008): 137.
12. R. Klein and R. Armitage, "Rhythms in Human Performance: 1½-Hour Oscillations in Cognitive Style," *Science* 204 (1979): 1326–28.
13. Guru Prem Singh Khalsa, *Divine Alignment: The Grace of Kundalini Yoga* (Beverly Hills, CA: Cherdi Kala Productions, 2005), 24.
14. D. Werntz, R. Bickford, F. Bloom, and D. Shannahoff-Khalsa, "Alternating Cerebral Hemispheric Activity and the Lateralization of Autonomic Nervous Function," *Human Neurobiology* 2 (1983): 39–43.
15. R. Klein, D. Pilon, S. Prosser, and D. Shannahoff-Khalsa, "Nasal Airflow Asymmetries and Human Performance," *Biological Psychology* 23 (1986): 127–137.
16. D. Werntz, R. Bickford, and D. Shannahoff-Khalsa, "Selective Hemispheric Stimulation by Unilateral Forced Nostril Breathing," *Human Neurobiology* 6 (1987): 165–171.
17. S. Rao and A. Potdar, "Nasal Airflow with the Body in Various Positions," *Journal of Applied Psychology* 28 (1970): 162–165.
18. R. Sovik, "The Science of Breathing–The Yogic View," *Progressive Brain Research* 122 (2000): 491–505.
19. R. P. Brown and P. Gerbarg, "Sudarshan Kriya Yogic Breathing in the Treatment of Stress, Anxiety, and Depression: Part I–Neurophysiologic Model," *Journal of Alternative & Complementary Medicine* 11, no. 1 (February 2005): 189–201.
20. R. Jerath, J. W. Edry, V. A. Barnes, and V. Jerath, "Physiology of Long Pranayamic Breathing: Neural Respiratory Elements May Provide a Mechanism That Explains How Slow Deep Breathing Shifts the Autonomic Nervous System," *Medical Hypotheses* 67 (2006): 566–571.

21. E. Nelson and J. Panksepp, "Brain Substrates of Infant-Mother Attachment: Contributions of Opioids, Oxytocin, and Norepinephrine," *Neuroscience Biobehavioral Review* 22 (1998): 437–452.

22. A. Frasch, T. Zetzche, A. Steiger, and G. F. Jirikowski, "Reduction of Plasma Oxytocin Levels in Patients Suffering from Major Depression," *Advances in Experimental Medicine and Biology* 1, no. 395 (1995): 257–258.

23. K. E. Habib, P. Gold, and G. P. Chrousos, "Neuroendocrinology of Stress," *Endocrinology Metabolism Clinics of North America* 30 (2001): 695–728.

24. C. Tsingos and G. P. Chrousos, "Hypothalamic-Pituitary-Adrenal Axis, Neuroendocrine Factors and Stress," *Journal of Psychosomatic Research* 53 (2002): 865–871.

Component 6: Snooze to Surge

1. Susan Yara, "Ten Ways to Sleep Better," Forbes.com, http://www.forbes.com/health/2005/09/06/insomnia-executivehealth-lifestyle-cx_sy_0907feat_Is.html (September 7, 2005).

2. Lawrence Epstein, *Improving Sleep: A Guide to a Good Night's Rest* (Cambridge, MA: Harvard Medical Publications, 2007), 48.

3. "You Snooze, You Lose? Looking for Links between Sleep, Appetite and Obesity," *Tufts University Health & Nutrition Letter* (April 2005): 6.

4. National Sleep Foundation, "Hungry for Sleep," *Fitness Matters* 11, Issue 5 (September-October 2005): 11.

5. Ibid.

6. Liz Neporent, "You Snooze, You Lose?," *Prevention*, 58 (March 2006): 33.

7. National Sleep Foundation, "Hungry for Sleep."

8. "Wake Up to More Muscle," *Men's Health* (April 2008): 52.

9. PsychCentral.com, "Too Much, Too Little Sleep Linked to Obesity, Smoking," http://psychcentral.com/news/2008/05/08/too-much-too-little-sleep-linked-to-obesity-smoking/2252.html (May 8, 2008).

10. CNN.com, "Sleep Deprivation as Bad as Alcohol Impairment, Study Suggests," http://archives.cnn.com/2000/HEALTH/09/20/sleep.deprivation (September 2000).

11. CBS News, "The Science of Sleep," http://cbsnews.com/stories/2008/03/14/60minutes/main3939721.shtml?source=search_story (March 14, 2008).

12. Allison Avery, "Why You Really Need Your Beauty Sleep," *Health Magazine* (January-February 2008): 150.

13. Heather Loeb, "Is Sleep Really Necessary?" *Men's Health* (June 2008): 137.

14. Gene Emery, "Heart Attack Risk Shifted by Daylight Saving Time," Reuters.com, http://www.reuters.com/article/lifestyleMolt/idUSTRE49T6DO20081030 (October 30, 2008).

15. Heather Loeb, "Is Sleep Really Necessary?"

16. Physorg.com, "Both Short and Long Sleep Is Associated with Increased Mortality," http://www.physorg.com/news110455029.html (October 1, 2007).

17. "The Guide to a Good Night's Sleep," *Health Magazine* (January-February 2008): 160.

18. National Sleep Foundation, "Hungry for Sleep."

19. PsychCentral.com, "Too Much, Too Little Sleep Linked to Obesity, Smoking."

20. Physorg.com, "Both Short and Long Sleep Is Associated with Increased Mortality."

21. N. Buscemi, B. Vandermeer, C. Friesen, L. Bialy, M. Tubman, M. Ospina, T. P. Klassen, and M. Witmans, "Manifestations and Management of Chronic Insomnia in Adults," Evidence Report/Technology Assessment: Number 125, http://www.ahrq.gov/clinic/epcsums/insomnsum.htm.

22. Ripu D. Jindal, Daniel J. Buysse, and Michael E. Thase, "Maintenance Treatment of Insomnia: What Can We Learn from the Depression Literature?" *American Journal of Psychiatry* 161 (January 2004): 19–24.

23. "The Bed of Your Dreams," *Health Magazine* (January-February 2008): 157.

24. Kim Bergoldt et al, "Better Backs by Better Beds?" *Spine* 33, no. 7 (April 2008): 703–708.
25. Woodson Merrell, "Your Best Energy Source–Sound Sleep," *O, The Oprah Magazine* (October 2008): 171.
26. Mayoclinic.org, "Dog Tired? It Could Be Your Pooch," https://www.mayoclinic.org/news2002-rst/954.html (February 14, 2002).
27. Mayoclinic.com, "Insomnia: Coping and Support" http://www.mayoclinic.com/health/insomnia/DS00187/DSECTION=coping-and-support (March 16, 2007).
28. Ibid.
29. "Bed Bugged," *Women's Health* (December 2007): 22.
30. Sally Wadka, "Either . . . OR?" *Real Simple* (August 2005): 77–78.
31. Nancy Gottesman, "Why You Really Need Your Beauty Rest," *O, The Oprah Magazine* (May 2008): 196.
32. Lee Ferris et al, "Resistance Training Improves Sleep Quality in Older Subjects," *Journal of Sports Science and Medicine* 14, no. 3 (2005): 354–360.
33. Nancy McVicar, "Doctors Advise against Reliance on Sleeping Pills for a Good Night's Rest," *South Florida Sun-Sentinel*, http://www.ajc.com/health/content/health/stories/001706sleep.html (January 15, 2006).
34. Ryan English, "Insomnia and Pregnancy," Ezine Articles, http://ezinearticles.com/?Insomnia-and-Pregnancy&id=1589494.
35. Natural Medicines Comprehensive Database, "Valerian," www.naturaldatabase.com (July 5, 2007).
36. Natural Standard Database, "Valerian," www.naturalstandard.com (July 3, 2007).
37. N. Little, "Natural Sleep Aids: Herbs and Vitamins for Sleep Difficulty," *Insight Journal,* http://www.anxiety-and-depressionsolutions.com/wellness_concerns/sleep/herbs_and_vitamins_for_sleep_difficulty.php (January 1, 2007).
38. Holisticonline.com, "Alternative and Integral Therapies for Insomnia," http://holisticonline.com/Remedies/Sleep/sleep_insomnia_alt_therapies.htm.
39. N. Little, "Natural Sleep Aids: Herbs and Vitamins for Sleep Difficulty."
40. Ibid.
41. Ibid.
42. "Cell Phone Use May Lead to Insomnia," Prognosis E-News, Wayne State University, http://www.metromodemedia.com/inthenews/cellstudy0052.aspx (January 24, 2008).
43. J. Lumeng, D. Somashekar, D. Appugliese, N. Kaciroti, R. Corwyn, and R. Bradley, "Shorter Sleep Duration Is Associated with Increased Risk for Being Overweight at Ages 9 to 12 Years," *Pediatrics* 120, no. 5 (November 2007): 1020–29.

Component 7: Mind-Set to Surge

1. Ernest L. Rossi, *The Psychobiology of Gene Expression* (New York: Norton, 2002), 65.
2. Ernest Rossi, *A Discourse with our Genes* (Benevento, Italy: Editris Press, 2005), 27.
3. C. Wrosch, G. E. Miller, M. F. Scheier, and S. Brun de Pontet, "Giving Up on Unattainable Goals: Benefits for Health?" *Personality and Social Psychology Bulletin* 33 (2007): 251–265.
4. H. R. Hall, "Hypnosis and the Immune System," *American Journal of Clinical Hypnosis* 25, no. 2–3 (1982–1983): 92–103.
5. G. Kolata, "Runner's High? Endorphins? Fiction, Some Scientists Say," *New York Times*, May 21, 2002, F1, F6.
6. N. E. Rosenthal, *The Emotional Revolution: How the New Science of Feelings Can Transform Your Life* (New York: Citadel Press Books, 2002), 330–331, 335.
7. Guang Yue and K. J. Cole, "Strength Increases from the Motor Program: Comparison of Training with Maximal Voluntary and Imagined Muscle Contractions," *Journal of Neurophysiology* 67, no. 5 (1992): 1114–23.
8. "Laugh Away Stress, Improve Your Mind," *Scientific American Mind* (June-July 2008): 9.
9. Chris C. Streeter, J. Eric Jensen, Ruth M. Perlmutter, Howard J. Cabral, Hua Tian, Devin B. Terhune, Domenic A. Ciraulo, and Perry F. Renshaw, "Yoga Asana Sessions Increase Brain GABA Levels: A Pilot Study," *The Journal of Alternative and Complementary Medicine* (May 2007): 419–426.

10. Richard P. Brown and Patricia L. Gerbarg, "Sudarshan Kriya Yogic Breathing in the Treatment of Stress, Anxiety, and Depression: Part I—Neurophysiologic Model," *Journal of Alternative and Complementary Medicine* 11, no. 1 (February 2005): 189–201.

11. Nikolai A. Shevchuk, "Adapted Cold Shower as a Potential Treatment for Depression," *Medical Hypotheses* 70, no. 5 (2008): 995–1001.

12. Oohoi.com, "Water Therapy Effectiveness," *Clinical Studies of Water Therapy*, http://www.oohoi.com/physical_therapy/water_therapy/effectiveness.htm.

13. Nancy Rones, "Your Guide to Never Feeling Tired Again," WebMD, http://www.webmd.com/balance/features/your-guide-to-never-feeling-tired-again? (December 3, 2008).

14. G. Rein, M. Atkinson, and R. McCraty, "The Physiological and Psychological Effects of Compassion and Anger," *Journal of Advancement in Medicine* 8, no. 2 (1995): 87–105.

Component 8: De-Stress to Surge

1. Uft Lundberg, "Stress, Subjective and Objective Health," *International Journal of Social Welfare* 15 (2006): 41–48.

2. Jeff Autor Gee and Val Autor Gee, "The Winner's Attitude: Change How You Deal with Difficult People and Get the Best Out of Any Situation," McNeil & Johnson (2006): 140

3. Mark A. Hyman, "Refrigerator Rights: The Missing Link in Health, Disease and Obesity," *Alternative Therapies in Health and Medicine* 4, no. 11 (2005): 10–12.

4. Megan Gunnar and Karina Quevedo, "The Neurobiology of Stress and Development," *Annual Review of Psychology* 58 (January 2007): 145–170.

5. PreventDisease.com, "Stop Being Tired: 20 Lifestyle Changes That Ensure Optimal Energy Levels," http://preventdisease.com/home/weeklywellness345.shtml (October 8, 2007).

6. The Independent, "Arggh! Who Says I'm Stressed?" http://www.independent.co.uk/news/media/arggh-who-says-im-stressed-754061.html (December 13, 2004).

7. "How Much Stress Does It Take to Make a Man Go Grey?," *Best Life* (October 2008): 20.

8. A. Steptoe et al, "The Effects of Tea on Psychophysiological Stress Responsivity and Post-Stress Recovery," *Journal of Psychopharmacology* 190, no. 1 (January 2007): 81–89.

9. Medical News Today, "Chewing Gum May Help Reduce Stress According to New Research," www.medicalnewstoday.com/articles/119826.php (September 1, 2008).

10. M. M. Delmonte, "Meditation and Anxiety Reduction: A Literature Review," *Clinical Psychology Review* 5 (1985): 91–102.

11. Sarah Lasar, "Meditation and Mindfulness Are in the National News," *Cape Stress Reduction & Optimal Health Newsletter* 11, no. 1 (March 2006): 1.

12. Robert H. Schneider, Kenneth G. Walton, John W. Salerno, and Sanford I. Nidich, "Cardiovascular Disease Prevention and Health Promotion with the Transcendental Meditation Program and Maharishi Consciousness-Based Health Care," *Ethnicity & Disease* 16 (3 Suppl 4): S4–15–26.

13. Judith Viorst, *Imperfect Control: Our Lifelong Struggles with Power and Surrender* (New York: Simon and Schuster, 1999), 205–236.

14. Deepak Chopra, *Quantum Healing: Exploring the Frontiers of Mind/Body Medicine* (New York: Bantam Books, 1989), 194.

15. Ibid.

16. Robert K. Wallace and Herbert Benson, "A Wakeful Hypometabolic Physiologic State," *American Journal of Physiology* 221, no. 3 (September 1971): 795–99.

17. R. J. Davidson, R.J. Kabat-Zinn, et al, "Meditation and Change in the Brain," *Psychosomatic Medicine* 65 (2003): 564–70.

18. Donna Eden, *Energy Medicine* (London: Piatkus Books, 1998), 278–279.

19. National Institutes of Health, *Acupuncture: NIH Consensus Statement* (Washington, DC: National Institutes of Health, 1997), 1–34.

20. Roger Callahan, *Stop the Nightmares of Trauma: Thought Field Therapy, the Power Therapy for the 21st Century* (Chapel Hill, NC: Professional Press, 2000), 231–251.
21. Judith A. Sutherland, "Getting to the Point," *American Journal of Nursing* 100, no. 9 (September 2000): 40.
22. S. Marcus, P. Marquis, and C. Sakai, "Controlled Study of Treatment of PTSD Using EMDR in an HMO Setting," *Psychotherapy* 34 (1997): 307–15.
23. Kathi Kemper and Suzanne C. Danhauer, "Music as Therapy," *Southern Medical Journal* 98, no. 3 (March 2005): 282–86.
24. Daniel L. Levitin, *This Is Your Brain on Music* (New York: Dutton, 2006), 180–183.

Component 9: Music Appreciation 101 to Surge

1. A. W. Harvey, "Utilizing Music as a Tool for Healing," in R. Pratt, ed., *The Fourth International Symposium on Music: Rehabilitation and Well-being* (Lanham, MD: University Press of America, 1987), 73–87.
2. A. W. Harvey, "On Developing a Program in Music Medicine: A Neurophysiological Basis for Music as Therapy," in R. Spingte and R. Droh, eds., *MusicMedicine* (St. Louis: MMB Music, 1992), 71–79.
3. Kathi J. Kemper and Suzanne C. Danhauer, "Music as Therapy," *Southern Medical Journal* 98, no. 3 (March 2005): 282–86.
4. Susan Hallam, "The Power of Music," http://musiced.org.uk/teachers/powerofmusic/index.html.
5. R. Abdollahanjad, "English Abstracts of the 4th Congress on Music Application in Mental and Physical Health, May 26–29, 2004," *Music Therapy Today* VI, no. 1 (February 2005): 96–112.
6. Baltimore Hospital, "Healing Aspects of Music Physically and Medicinally," http://cc.ysu.edu/~s0133456/healing_aspects_of_music_physically.htm.
7. Robert E. Krout, "Music Listening to Facilitate Relaxation and Promote Wellness: Integrated Aspects of Our Neurophysiological Responses to Music," *The Arts in Psychotherapy* 34 (2007): 134–141.
8. Barry Bittman, "Playing a Musical Instrument Reverses Stress on the Genomic Level," http://www.medicalnewstoday.com/articles/19535.php (May 22, 2007).
9. R. Kopiez, A. C. Lehmann, I. Wolther, and C. Wolf, "Does Singing Provide Health Benefits?" Proceedings of the 5th Triennial ESCOM Conference September 8–13, 2003, Hanover University of Music and Drama, Germany.
10. C. Conrad, H. Niess, K. W. Jauch, C. J. Bruns, W. Hartl, and L. Welker, "Overture for Growth Hormone: Requiem for Interleukin-6," *Critical Care Medicine* 35 (2007): 2709–13.
11. Ann Readapt, "Effect of Music Therapy among Hospitalized Patients with Chronic Low Back Pain: A Controlled, Randomized Trial," *Medical Physics* 48, no. 5 (June 2005): 217–224.
12. *Men's Health,* "The Science of Workout Music," http://www.menshealth.com/cda/article.do?site=MensHealth&channel=fitness&category=music.on.the.go&conitem=d9b85ae142396010VgnVCM100000cfe793cd__.
13. U. Nilsson, M. Unosson, and N. Rawal, "Stress Reduction and Analgesia in Patients Exposed to Calming Music Postoperatively: A Randomized Controlled Trial," *European Journal of Anaesthesiology* 22 (2005): 96–102.
14. *Men's Health*, "The Science of Workout Music," op cit, no. 10, above.
15. Robert E. Krout, "Music Listening to Facilitate Relaxation and Promote Wellness."
16. Marjan Farshadi and Moigan Farshadi, "Investigation of Effects of Music Therapy in Reducing Sleep Disorders in High School Girls," *Music Therapy Today* VI, no. 1 (February 2005): 110–111.
17. "Music in Stroke Rehabilitation," *The Lancet* 371, no. 9614 (February 2008): 698.
18. *Men's Health*, "The Science of Workout Music," page 238.
19. Susan Hallum, "The Power of Music," http://musiced.org.uk/teachers/powerofmusic/index.html.
20. Smartkit, "Music Training Can Remodel the Brainstem and Improve Learning," http://www.smart-kit.com/index.php?s=Mozart (March 25, 2007).
21. Noel Geoghegan and Janine McCaffrey, "The Impact of Music Education on Children's Overall Development: Towards a

Proactive Advocacy," *Australian Association for Research in Music Education, Proceedings of the XXVIth Annual Conference*, September 25–28, 2004, 163–176.
22. Lee Crust and Peter J. Clough, "The Influence of Rhythm and Personality in the Endurance Response to Motivational Asynchronous Music," *Journal of Sports Sciences* 24, no. 2 (February 2006): 187–195.
23. J. M. Standley, "A Meta-analysis of the Efficacy of Music Therapy for Premature Infants," *Journal of Pediatric Nursing* 17, no. 2 (2002): 107–113.
24. J. Stouffer, B. Shirk, and R. Polomano, "Practice Guidelines for Music Interventions with Hospitalized Pediatric Patients," *Journal of Pediatric Nursing* 24, no. 6 (1998): 532–38.
25. Christine Larson, "The Fine Art of Healing the Sick: Embracing the Benefits of Writing, Music, and Art," *U.S. News and World Report*, June 5, 2006, 3.
26. Reuters.com. "Slow Eating Trims Calorie Intake: Study," http://www.reuters.com/article/healthNews/idUSCOL85478620080708 (July 8, 2008).
27. Patricia Ambroziak, "Tune in Boo! Use Music to Improve Health and Performance," *American Fitness* (September-October 2003): 29–31.
28. Joe Verghese, Richard B. Lipton, Mindy J. Katz, et al, "Leisure Activities and the Risk of Dementia in the Elderly," *New England Journal of Medicine* 348, no. 25 (June 19, 2003): 2508–16.
29. Miranda Hitti, "Dancing Your Way to Better Health," FoxNews.com, http://www.foxnews.com/story/0,2933,160965,00.html (June 29, 2005).

Component 10: Sex to Big *Surge*

1. time.com, Anastasia Toufexis, Hannah Bloch, and Sally B. Donnelly, "The Right Chemistry," http://www.time.com/time/magazine/article/0.9171.977754-1.00.html (February 15, 1993).
2. Wikipedia, "Pheromone," http://en.wikipedia.org/wiki/Pheromone.
3. K. Grammer and A. Jütte, "Battle of Odors: Significance of Pheromones for Human Reproduction," Pubmed.gov, http://www.ncbi.nlm.nih.gov/pubmed/9483874
4. James McBride Dabbs, *Heroes, Rogues, and Lovers: Testosterone and Behavior* (New York: McGraw-Hill, 2000), 24–38.
5. Helen Fisher, *Why We Love* (New York. Henry Holt: 2004), 52–53.
6. Ibid.
7. BBC News, "Sex Chemistry 'Lasts Two Years,'" http://news.bbc.co.uk/1/hi/health/4669104.stm (February 1, 2006).
8. Helen Fisher, *Why We Love*, 52–53.
9. Douglas A. Granger, Alan Booth, and David R. Johnson, "Human Aggression and Enumerative Measures of Immunity," *Psychosomatic Medicine* 62 (2000): 583–590.
10. cbsnews.com, "Top 10 Reasons to Have Sex Tonight and More Sex," http://www.cbsnews.com/stories/2008/...n3962093.shtml (March 24, 2008).
11. Ibid.
12. Lauren Cox, "Headaches and Sex: 'Yes, Tonight Dear,'" ABC News, http://abcnews.go.com/Health/PainManagement/Story?id=4241193&page=1= (February 5, 2008).
13. J. Koskimäki, R. Shiri, T. Tammela, J. Häkkinen, M. Hakama, and A. Auvinen, "Regular Intercourse Protects Against Erectile Dysfunction: Tampere Aging Male Urologic Study. Preview," *American Journal of Medicine*, July 2008, 121, issue 7, 592–596..
14. Helen Fisher, page 239.
15. Todd Neale, "Many Women with Sexual Dysfunction Simply Don't Care," MedPage Today, http://www.medpagetoday.com/OBGYN/GeneralOBGYN/11574 (October 31, 2008).
16. Dance with Shadows, "Diet Can Help Women Boost Low Libido," http://www.dancewithshadows.com/business/pharma/diet-women-libido.asp (May 4, 2007).

17. Sharon Krum, "The Raging Libido Diet," *London Times*, January 17, 2004, http://www.naturalnurse.com/raginglabido.htm.
18. Forbes.com, "The Better Sex Diet," http://www.forbes.com/2006/12/05/leadership-health-sex-lead-innovation-cx_tw_1205sex.html (December 5, 2006).
19. Ray Burton, Risingwomen.com "How is Your Libido? What to Do About A Drop in Libido," http://www.risingwomen.com/Jan%202005%20health%20burton.htm (January 20, 2005).
20. Ibid.
21. Colette Bouchez, "Better Sex: What's Weight Got to Do with It?" WebMD, http://www.webmd.com/sex-relationships/guide/sex-and-weight (March 25, 2005).
22. National Women's Health Report, "Midlife Women and Sexual Health," www.wiawh.org/media/document/pdf/National WomensHealthReport%20Midlife.pdf (April 2005).
23. Danna Schneider, "Kegels for Childbirth and More," Natural Childbirth, http://childbirth.amuchbetterway.com/kegels-for-childbirth-and-more/
24. Netdoctor, "Pelvic Floor Exercises," http://www.netdoctor.co.uk/womenshealth/sui/pelvicfloor_005167.htm (March 22, 2005).
25. National Association for Continence, "Pelvic Muscle Exercises," http://www.nafc.org/bladder-bowel-health/types-of-incontinence/stress-incontinence/pelvic-muscle-exercises.
26. Guru Prem Singh Khalsa, *Divine Alignment: The Grace of Kundalini Yoga*, (Beverly Hills: Cherdi Kala Productions, 2003), 1.
27. Laurie B. Rosenblum, MPH, "Sex After Menopause," https://healthlibrary.epnet.com/GetContent.aspx?token=0d429707-b7ei-4147-9947-abca6797a602&chunkiid=14512
28. Ibid.
29. Amy Levin-Epstein, "Seven Powerful Penis Foods," *Best Life* (August 2008): 72.
30. "Fit for Baby Making," *Women's Health* (December 2008): 32.
31. S. Gold, "A Higher Road to Relaxation," *Psychology Today* 40, 4 (July 1, 2007): 57–58.
32. Chip Walter, "Affairs of the Lips," *Scientific American Mind* 19, no. 1 (February-March 2008): 24–29.
33. Deborah P. Welsh, Peter T. Haugen, Laura Widman, Nancy Darling, and Catherine M. Grello, "Kissing Is Good: A Developmental Investigation of Sexuality in Adolescent Romantic Couples," *Journal of Sexuality Research and Social Policy* 2 (December 2005): 32–41.
34. Ibid.
35. C. Walter, "Affairs of the Lips," 24–29.
36. A. Aron, C. Norman, C. McKenna, and R. E. Heyman, "Couples' Shared Participation in Novel and Arousing Activities and Experienced Relationship Quality," *Journal of Personality and Social Psychology* 78, no. 2 (2000): 273–84.
37. Nancy Rones, "Your Guide to Never Feeling Tired Again," WebMD, http://www.webmd.com/balance/features/your-guide-to-never-feeling-tired-again (December 3, 2008).
38. E. Harburg, N. Kaciroti, L. Gleiberman, M. Julius, M. Schork, "Marital Pair Anger-Coping Types May act as an Entity to Affect Mortality: Preliminary Findings from a Prospective Study," *Journal of Family Communication*, 8 (2008) : 44–61.
39. Allison Van Dusen, "How to Make Your Spouse Live Longer," Forbes.com, http://www.forbes.com/health/2008/02/04/health-spouse-life-forbeslife-cx_avd_0204health.html (February 2008).

Conclusion

1. Justnews.com. Tony Cappasso, "Go to Church, Live Longer," http://www.justnews.com/sh/health/dailytips/health-dailytips-20000127-231757.html (March 30, 2001)
2. Peggy Thoits, Ann A. Hohmann, Mary R. Harvey, and Bill Fletcher, "Volunteer Work and Well-being," *Journal of Health and Social Behavior* 42:(2001): 115–131

INDEX

Boldface page references indicate photographs or illustrations. Underscored references indicate boxed text and charts.

C

F

M

N

O

T

U

V